100 Questions & Answers About Attention-Deficit Hyperactivity Disorder (ADHD) in Women and Girls

Patricia O. Quinn, MD
Director
National Center for Girls and Women with AD/HD
Washington, DC

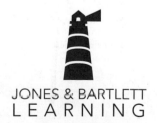

JONES & BARTLETT
LEARNING

World Headquarters
Jones & Bartlett Learning
40 Tall Pine Drive
Sudbury, MA 01776
978-443-5000
info@jblearning.com
www.jblearning.com

Jones & Bartlett Learning
Canada
6339 Ormindale Way
Mississauga, Ontario L5V 1J2
Canada

Jones & Bartlett Learning
International
Barb House, Barb Mews
London W6 7PA
United Kingdom

Jones & Bartlett Learning books and products are available through most bookstores and online booksellers. To contact Jones & Bartlett Learning directly, call 800-832-0034, fax 978-443-8000, or visit our website, www.jblearning.com.

Substantial discounts on bulk quantities of Jones & Bartlett Learning publications are available to corporations, professional associations, and other qualified organizations. For details and specific discount information, contact the special sales department at Jones & Bartlett Learning via the above contact information or send an email to specialsales@jblearning.com.

The authors, editor, and publisher have made every effort to provide accurate information. However, they are not responsible for errors, omissions, or for any outcomes related to the use of the contents of this book and take no responsibility for the use of the products and procedures described. Treatments and side effects described in this book may not be applicable to all people; likewise, some people may require a dose or experience a side effect that is not described herein. Drugs and medical devices are discussed that may have limited availability controlled by the Food and Drug Administration (FDA) for use only in a research study or clinical trial. Research, clinical practice, and government regulations often change the accepted standard in this field. When consideration is being given to use of any drug in the clinical setting, the healthcare provider or reader is responsible for determining FDA status of the drug, reading the package insert, and reviewing prescribing information for the most up-to-date recommendations on dose, precautions, and contraindications, and determining the appropriate usage for the product. This is especially important in the case of drugs that are new or seldom used.

Production Credits
Executive Publisher: Christopher Davis
Editorial Assistant: Sara Cameron
Associate Production Editor: Laura Almozara
Associate Marketing Manager: Katie Hennessy
Manufacturing and Inventory Supervisor: Amy Bacus
Composition: Glyph International
Cover Design: Carolyn Downer
Cover Images: Top left photo: © Tracy Whiteside/ShutterStock, Inc.; Top right photo:
    © Juice Team/ShutterStock, Inc.; Bottom photo: © Tyler Olson/ShutterStock, Inc.
Printing and Binding: Malloy, Inc.
Cover Printing: Malloy, Inc.

Library of Congress Cataloging-in-Publication Data
Quinn, Patricia O.
   100 questions & answers about attention-deficit hyperactivity disorder
(ADHD) in women and girls / Patricia Quinn.
      p. cm.
   Includes bibliographical references and index.
   ISBN 978-0-7637-8452-2 (alk. paper)
   1. Attention-deficit disorder in adults—Popular works. 2.
Attention-deficit disorder in adolescence—Popular works. 3. Women—Mental
health. 4. Teenage girls—Mental health. I. Title. II. Title: One hundred
questions and answers about attention-deficit hyperactivity disorder (ADHD)
in women and girls.
   RC394.A85Q85 2012
   616.85'890082—dc22

                                                                2010032213

6048

Printed in the United States of America
14 13 12 11 10   10 9 8 7 6 5 4 3 2 1

Contents

Our understanding of ADHD has changed so profoundly over the past several decades that much of what we understand about it today was completely unknown in the late 1960s when I received my initial clinical training. It's been an exciting and fascinating journey, participating in the explosion of knowledge about the brain and how it functions. Closer to home, however, it has been a particularly important journey, as I gradually came to recognize my own ADHD (which certainly didn't fit our understanding of hyperkinesis in the 1960s) and worked to help my daughter with ADHD to get the assistance and support that would never have been available to her had she been born a generation earlier.

In those long-ago days, we believed all sorts of things about the brain that we now know are not true. The condition we now know as ADHD (attention-deficit hyperactivity disorder) was called "minimal brain dysfunction" or "hyperkinesis." We observed very hyperactive, impulsive young boys who tended to function poorly in school. Because these boys typically became less hyperactive after puberty, we mistakenly thought that they had outgrown their disorder. What we now know is that adolescence marks the beginning of even greater challenges for those growing up with ADHD.

What we didn't know then was that hyperactivity wasn't the core of the problem—it was simply the most noticeable symptom. Later, in the 1980s, a revolution in our thinking took place when it was recognized that nonhyperactive children also had problems with inattention and distractibility. And with this recognition, the name changed to ADD (attention-deficit disorder). This shift cracked open the door a tiny bit to allow more girls to be diagnosed. Over the years, the reported ratio of boys to girls diagnosed with ADHD gradually shifted from 9:1 down to 3:1, but stubbornly remained there for more than 20 years.

As I continued in my career, I was also in the process of raising my daughter. Because she was more hyperactive than many girls, her pediatrician mentioned the likelihood of ADHD when she was a preschooler. Just a few minutes of observing her fidgeting and squirming on the examination table and noting her little legs decorated with an array of bruises from all of her exploratory tree climbing caught his attention. Although my daughter was first diagnosed in the mid-1970s, this early diagnosis did her little good. School programs to help those with ADHD remained far in the future, and even today, few public schools have adequate supports or programs in place to meet the needs of girls. Along with other mothers of similar daughters, I worked to cobble together a support system that wasn't available in the public schools—counselors and tutors—which helped, but not enough to make school an enjoyable experience for my very bright child.

Meanwhile, I continued to work with many children, adolescents, and their families. I was very familiar with the male version of the disorder. My younger brother had exhibited classic symptoms. He was the little boy in the back of the class, bored, restless, frustrated, and paying more attention to looking for ways to pass the time until the school day ended than paying attention to class instruction.

The more I listened to my clients throughout the 1980s, the more a light began to dawn as I gradually came to recognize my own ADHD. I had never been a discipline problem for my parents and had been a good student, so my struggles were easy to overlook. But the more I learned about ADHD, the clearer it became—why I was such a tomboy, enjoying playing with my brothers more than engaging in passive female pastimes; why I had difficulty with handwriting; why I was always talking in class; and why I was a compulsive chair tipper despite countless warnings and admonishments. Aha! Finally I understood the incident in college when I was dropped off at the airport several hours early, yet still missed my plane because I'd lost track of time. Finally, it made sense to me why, although I was a good student, I always needed to ask a classmate about instructions that had just been explained to the entire class; why I never seemed to feel sleepy at bedtime; and why I planned at least twice too many tasks for each day.

Together, my daughter and I learned coping skills. I wrote reminders to myself on sticky notes, and soon my daughter was doing the same—posting messages to herself throughout the house to remind her to feed the cat.

Humor became one of the most important coping skills. I taught my daughter to laugh at her own struggles by telling tales about myself. One classic ADHD tale of mine was the morning that I left for the office, bringing a carton of my recently published first book. This book, now published by the American Psychological Association, was initially self-published for the benefit of clients at our clinic. I kept the stock of books at home and brought in a box as needed. On this particular morning, I placed the box of books on the top of my car in order to unlock the car door. Without benefit of my first cup of coffee (I was on my way to purchase it), I unwittingly left the box of books on the car top and drove several blocks to the neighborhood bagel shop. As I parked in front, the owner of the shop, who knew me well, came toward me laughing. "I think you forgot something," she teased. I looked up to find the box of books still, thankfully, on the roof of my car. Laughing with her, I exclaimed "You won't believe what's in that box!" It's a book called, *Learning to Slow Down and Pay Attention* (Magination Press, 1997). And, what's even worse, I wrote the book!" I yelped with laughter, appreciating the irony of the title, given what I'd just done.

I loved to share this story with my daughter as a great example of the unpredictability of living with ADHD—that I was capable of writing and publishing a book, yet not always capable of remembering that I'd put a box of those books on the top of my car.

As my daughter came to understand her own ADHD, she easily recognized ADHD patterns in some of her friends and was jokingly referred to as the "ADHD poster child." Unable to find the structure and support she needed in large public school classrooms, her struggles grew during middle and high school until she finally requested, in her sophomore year, to go away to a private boarding school where she would finally receive the assistance that would allow her to succeed in high school and go on to college. Students with ADHD in general, and girls with ADHD in particular, were not being well-served in the public school system or the professional community, where their ADHD was typically overlooked or misunderstood.

The awareness of ADHD in adults exploded following the publication of *Driven to Distraction* in 1995 (Touchstone)—a best-selling book that led to broad public awareness of ADHD in adults. Several adult ADHD clinics were opened across the United States, and women came in droves, self-referred, to explore whether their lifelong struggles had a name, an explanation, and a treatment. While this was still considered to be a primarily male disorder, in these new adult ADHD clinics, the male–female ratios were nearly 1:1! What could be going on to explain this huge difference?

The mid-1990s were a time of new revelations about ADHD. Right on the heels of *Driven to Distraction*, the first book on ADHD in women, Sari Solden's *Women with Attention Deficit Disorder*, was published by Underwood Books in 1995. It became clear that females were the greatest underserved ADHD population and Pat Quinn and I formed a partnership to focus our professional careers on ADHD in females and began to publish *ADDvance Magazine*—a publication exclusively for women struggling to understand and get help for their newly diagnosed condition.

These were exciting times for us. As women who had each spent our careers in the field of ADHD, we were particularly motivated to promote the recognition and diagnosis of women. We'd seen too many women struggle, only to be blamed for those struggles rather than diagnosed and properly treated. In 1999, we coauthored *Understanding Girls With AD/HD*. That book was followed in 2002 by two others, *Understanding Women With AD/HD* and *Gender Issues and AD/HD* (a book for professionals on the diagnosis and treatment of women). We'd come a long way, baby. Invitations for media events and interviews for magazine articles came pouring in as ADHD in girls and women suddenly became a hot topic.

In the decade since those heady times, the progress continued. More research has focused on females and many girls and women have been helped in the intervening years, and yet there is still so much to be done. A troubling recent study showed that when teachers read identical anecdotes describing a student with ADHD symptoms—one anecdote with a girl's name attached and an identical anecdote with a boy's name attached—teachers report that they would be much more likely to refer the boy for evaluation and assistance.

In my clinical practice, it remains all too common for a woman to seek an assessment for ADHD at her own initiation after being treated for years for anxiety or depression with no recognition of possible ADHD. For women, ADHD remains the only psychiatric disorder I'm aware of in which the sufferers of the disorder are working to educate the professionals who treat them.

Oddly, it seems that public awareness has outpaced professional awareness. Now that we women know that we struggle with issues related to ADHD, the next stage is to educate professionals—teachers, professors, physicians, psychotherapists—still caught in old ways of thinking. And so the work goes on.

Kathleen Nadeau, PhD
Director, Chesapeake ADHD
Center of Maryland

Foreword

In 1969, when I wrote my first paper on attention-deficit hyperactivity disorder (ADHD), it was called minimal brain dysfunction, and I had no idea that I was embarking on a journey that would last for over 40 years. However, I do remember that I was instantly fascinated when I learned that alterations in the brain that could not even be seen by a microscope could cause behaviors, mainly hyperactivity and impulsivity, that could affect a person's functioning and wreak havoc in every aspect of her life. But, it was not until I read Dr. Paul Wender's book, *Minimal Brain Dysfunction in Children* (Wiley & Sons, 1971), which postulated a glitch in the monoamine system of the brain, mainly involving the neurotransmitters dopamine and norepinephrine and resulting in the hyperactivity observed in these children, that I was hooked.

From 1972 to 1974, I had the privilege of working with Dr. Judith Rapoport, a child psychiatrist, who, along with Drs. Wender, Cantwell, and Conners, was one of the pioneers in the ADHD movement. During my time with her, I honed my diagnostic skills by screening several hundred elementary school-aged boys for "hyperactivity syndrome" and conducted research on the effectiveness of various medications as treatments for ADHD.

In private practice and during my work as a consultant for many schools, I've worked with thousands of children and adults with ADHD, and they have all taught me a great deal. Many of my first patients were very hyperactive little boys, who despite their best efforts had great difficulty conforming to the standards of behavior expected in most elementary schools of the day. I learned how difficult it is to parent a child with ADHD and the strain that the disorder can place on the fabric of most families. I saw a few girls early on, but they all looked just like the little boys—hyperactive and somewhat unruly—nothing new there!

Over the years, however, two aspects of my practice began to change. First, I began seeing girls coming to me for diagnosis during their junior or senior years in high school or as they encountered problems academically, some for the first time, in college. Second, I began to focus more on ADD without hyperactivity—the inattentive subtype as it is called today. It was then that I came to the overwhelming realization that there were just as many girls and women suffering silently with ADHD as there were boys and men. Yet these girls and women had gone undiagnosed for decades.

ADHD is, to say the least, a very heterogeneous disorder. Its presentations vary from individual to individual and can change over time depending on life circumstances. High IQ, extraordinary coping skills, and a supportive environment can mitigate its impact. But just as likely, an individual with ADHD will have difficulty living up to his or her potential, resulting in overwhelming shame, demoralization, and an exquisite sense of being different from others. Failures in academic, social, or occupational domains take a heavy economic as well as emotional toll. Coexisting conditions such as depression, anxiety, oppositional defiant disorder, and learning disabilities are the norm rather than the exception, and yet, despite all of this dysfunction, individuals can triumph despite their ADHD.

Females with ADHD, however, pay the additional price of having gender role expectations placed on them by a society that has no equivalent of "boys will be boys" for girls with ADHD. ADHD traits of high activity level, competition, aggression, and risk taking are all seen as more negative in girls. Women are expected to be organized, to play by the rules, to be good at remembering countless details, and to meet others' needs before their own. Facing these impossible demands, women and girls with ADHD habitually become their own harshest critics. They characteristically internalize these feelings of negative self-worth, self-doubt, and helplessness and develop an internal dialog with negative scripts that undermine and thwart their efforts at success—all the while presenting a façade of competence covering the internal chaos and silent suffering. As a result, they hide their symptoms and repeatedly feel like imposters as they struggle valiantly, living a life that they sense they don't deserve. And when things don't turn out the way they had hoped, they feel justified and condemned to future failure.

But with knowledge comes power. By taking a look at ADHD through a different lens, not that of elementary school-aged boys or hyperactive boys grown up, the stories of women with ADHD were uncovered. Women like Sari Solden, Kathleen Nadeau, Julia Rucklidge, Bonnie Kaplan, and Jeneva Ohan all helped paint the picture of the struggles of girls with ADHD or women who had gone undiagnosed until later in life. While there are indeed similarities between the genders and a phenotypic core of ADHD symptoms that affect both sexes, recent findings have uncovered the true severity of the disorder in females and suggest that we need to rethink the models used for both the diagnosis and treatment of ADHD in girls and women. It is hoped that this book will contribute to that knowledge and answer many of the questions that you might have about ADHD in women and girls.

Patricia O. Quinn, MD
Director, National Center for Girls and Women with AD/HD
Washington, DC

Preface

PART ONE

ADHD in Women and Girls: What Are the Differences?

What is the prevalence of ADHD in males versus females?

What are the most common symptoms of ADHD in females?

Are certain subtypes of ADHD more common in females?

More . . .

1. What is ADHD?

Attention-deficit hyperactivity disorder (ADHD) is a real, lifelong condition characterized by core symptoms of inattention, distractibility, impulsivity, and hyperactivity—although these are by no means the only problems a person with ADHD encounters. The disorder results in behaviors that affect almost every aspect of a person's life resulting in impaired functioning that commonly persists into adulthood. The **neurobiologic** basis for ADHD is thought to be the result of problems with the brain's **chemical neurotransmitters**, particularly **dopamine** and **norepinephrine**. Recent advances in technologies (**brain scans** and **imaging studies**) have helped to uncover several differences in the brains of people diagnosed with ADHD.

ADHD is present from birth (congenital) and **inherited** in most cases (see a discussion of the genetics of ADHD in Question 16). However, in most people, symptoms do not appear for several years. At younger ages, hyperactivity is the most commonly observed symptom. Inattentiveness and problems with organization and **executive functions** are not usually seen until much later as life's demands increase or symptoms overwhelm a person's ability to cope.

Over the life span, symptoms of ADHD may change. What first appears as out-of-seat behavior, daydreaming, and careless mistakes in childhood may become inner restlessness, failure to plan ahead, incomplete projects, and forgetfulness in adulthood. In general, women and girls with ADHD are less hyperactive and more inattentive than males with the disorder. For a girl with ADHD, symptoms may not affect her functioning for years if she receives a lot of support at home or at school, has a high IQ, or if she works hard and uses coping strategies. People with ADHD commonly demonstrate a mix of symptoms, however, and a girl or woman will be diagnosed with one of the various types of ADHD depending on her predominant symptom presentation.

2. How is ADHD diagnosed?

Despite the many recent technological advances for the diagnosis of various medical conditions, ADHD remains a diagnosis based purely on the presence of a set of behaviors or symptoms that are of such intensity that they significantly affect a person's ability to function on a day-to-day basis over a period of time. Although abnormalities in certain areas of the brain have been seen on scans in numerous research studies, these findings represent group differences from normal control values and are not currently available or valid to make the diagnosis of ADHD in individual cases. In addition, while **gene** abnormalities have been found to occur more often in people with ADHD and their families, genetic testing for ADHD cannot be obtained routinely.

Over the years, other neurologic, psychological, and educational tests have been used in an attempt to make the diagnosis of ADHD more objective, but these too, have met with little success. Poor performance on vigilance testing (also known as **continuous performance testing**), once thought to be a marker for the inattention and impulsivity of ADHD, has been found to be ineffective for the diagnosis of ADHD. This is particularly true for inattentive-only females who would concentrate for the test receiving a score within the average range. Thus producing a false negative result that missed the diagnosis. Researchers have also undertaken to analyze and categorize brain wave patterns seen on **electroencephalograms**, suggesting that certain ratios may be seen in those with ADHD, thus aiding in the diagnostic process. Although there has been some promising research using this tool for diagnosis, it has not gained widespread acceptance. As a result, a valid, objective, and readily available test for making the diagnosis of ADHD remains elusive.

ADHD continues to be a diagnosis made by a trained physician or mental health professional after a comprehensive evaluation including a structured interview, rating scales to document symptoms, and a complete medical assessment. To be accurately diagnosed with ADHD, a person is required to meet certain diagnostic criteria as determined by the **American Psychiatric Association (APA)** and listed in the ***Diagnostic and Statistical Manual of Mental Disorders*, Fourth Edition, Text Revision (DSM-IV-TR)** (2000). For a diagnosis of ADHD, these **criteria** require that a person must demonstrate at least six of nine symptoms of inattention, or at least six of nine symptoms of hyperactivity/impulsivity; that these symptoms must have been present for at least 6 months; and that some symptoms were present before the age of 7. In addition, the person must demonstrate some impairment from the symptoms in two or more settings (e.g., at school or work and at home), and there must be **clinically significant impairment** in social, academic, or occupational functioning. The final requirement for diagnosis states that symptoms may not be caused by another or coexisting condition.

Using these DSM-IV-TR criteria, a person may be diagnosed with one of three subtypes of ADHD. These subtypes include:

1. *Predominantly inattentive subtype (IA)*—In this subtype, the individual will have six or more symptoms of inattentiveness and/or fewer than six of the symptoms of hyperactivity/impulsivity.

2. *Predominantly hyperactive/impulsive subtype (H/I)*—In this subtype, the individual will demonstrate six or more symptoms of hyperactivity/ impulsivity and fewer than six symptoms of inattentiveness.

3. *Combined subtype (C)*—In this subtype, the individual will demonstrate six or more (out of nine) symptoms in both the inattentive and hyperactive/impulsive categories.

Assignment to one subtype of ADHD is, however, not fixed, and a woman or girl's diagnosis may change from one subtype to another depending on the primary symptoms she exhibits at that time. For example, a girl with combined subtype ADHD in childhood may be diagnosed as having the inattentive subtype in adolescence as her hyperactivity lessens or abates. Or, a primarily inattentive adolescent female may have her diagnosis change to combined subtype in adulthood as impulsivity appears or intensifies and significantly affects her decision making and other behaviors.

For many females, a delay in obtaining a diagnosis of ADHD may be a direct result of the insensitivity of these DSM-IV-TR criteria to the early signs and symptoms of the disorder in females. In certain instances, there seem to be actual differences in the course of the disorder in females with symptoms presenting or not causing impairments until much later. The APA has recognized the diagnostic problems inherent in DSM-IV-TR and has suggested several proposed changes in DSM-5 (APA, 2010), which is scheduled to be released

ADHD in Women and Girls: What Are the Differences?

in 2013. These proposed changes include maintaining the present criteria but without subtypes or discontinuing predominantly hyperactive/impulsive and predominantly inattentive subtypes. The DSM-5 panel is also entertaining the possibility of making changes to the current inattentive subtype by either creating a separate diagnosis of attention-deficit disorder (ADD) with the same inattention criteria that are present in DSM-IV-TR or retaining the current predominantly inattentive subtype, but requiring that no more than two hyperactivity criteria contribute to the diagnosis. (To read a more in-depth discussion of the diagnostic picture of ADHD in females, a critique of each diagnostic criterion of DSM-IV-TR, the reasons why each misses the mark or fails completely in identifying females with ADHD, and the proposed changes in DSM-5, see Appendix A of this book.)

3. What is the prevalence of ADHD in males versus females?

ADHD has been estimated to affect 4.4% of adults and 8.7% of children ages 8 to 15 years. However, not all of these individuals are *diagnosed*, and it seems that girls are diagnosed less often than boys. For many years, boys, regardless of the subtype of ADHD, were diagnosed 10 times more often than girls (10 boys for every 1 girl!), but recently this ratio has dropped to 2.5 or 3 to 1. Studies investigating gender ratios in adults with ADHD have found that this difference in *rates of diagnosis* for males and females may actually disappear in adulthood (Walker, 1999; Faraone et al., 2000) with diagnosis occurring more often in a ratio of 1:1. While there are no reliable figures on the numbers of women with ADHD, or the true male-to-female ratio of adults with ADHD, all reports strongly suggest that women with ADHD represent a more significant proportion of adults with ADHD than had been previously recognized. In many adult ADHD clinics today, the number of women equals or exceeds the number of men being seen. It is thought that the near equal numbers of males and females diagnosed with ADHD in adulthood is due to the fact that women are not dependent on others for the referral and that it reflects the true incidence of the disorder in childhood.

Girls with ADHD continue to be seen in significantly fewer numbers than boys with ADHD, most likely because they are dependent on others, mainly teachers and parents, for the referral to a professional for an evaluation of their symptoms. Studies by Jeneva Ohan and others have demonstrated a significant bias against the referral of girls by teachers and parents for evaluation of ADHD symptoms. To investigate this premise, Ohan and Visser (2009) presented identical vignettes for review by teachers and parents of children with high ADHD symptoms. Half of the participants read scenarios with boys' names and half read the same vignette but with a girl's name (e.g., Alexander vs. Alexandra, Eric vs. Erica). After reading the vignette, parents and teachers rated their likelihood of referring the child for services and how much benefit they expected from three types of services. Findings indicated that parents and teachers were both less likely to refer girls for services, not because they were less disruptive, but because they believed that services were less effective for girls. In addition, the girls with ADHD were only referred less often than any other vignette type (i.e., boys with ADHD only and with ADHD and disruptive behavior, and girls with ADHD and disruptive behavior). Therefore, in gen-

Girls with ADHD continue to be seen in significantly fewer numbers than boys with ADHD.

eral, for girls who are referred, it is more likely that they demonstrate more severe symptoms and that these girls are not representative of the larger sample of girls in the general population who continue to suffer silently without a diagnosis.

4. What are the most common symptoms of ADHD in females?

The main symptoms of ADHD as defined by the DSM-IV-TR criterion are the same for males and females—inattentiveness, impulsivity, and **hyperactivity**. However, these symptoms may have different ways of presenting themselves in females, who are in general, less hyperactive and more inattentive. Overall, females tend to have fewer symptoms as measured by DSM-IV-TR, but they tend to be just as impaired as males by these symptoms. In addition, for some time it has been known that women and girls with ADHD are more likely to **internalize** their symptoms, saying things like: "I'm stupid" or "I can't do anything right." They are easily embarrassed and humiliated by the consequences of their ADHD symptoms and behaviors. They then become anxious that these same situations will occur again or depressed that things are not going well. In addition, women and girls with ADHD report that they suffer many daily ups and downs, often feeling like they are on an emotional roller coaster and that they have little or no control over their emotions (emotional dysregulation) in addition to their ADHD symptoms.

A study using the Wender Utah rating scale found interesting differences in ADHD symptoms as reported by men and women (Stein et al., 1995). Symptoms of ADHD most often reported by women were **dysphoria**, inattention, organization problems, and impulsive behaviors. Dysphoria, as reported in this study, was described as a reactive moodiness rather than true **depression**. By contrast, males reported more conduct problems, learning problems, stress intolerance, attention problems, and poor social skills. Important differences can also be found between males and females on self-ratings, where women usually report a poorer self-concept, fewer assets, and more problems than those reported by their male counterparts.

5. What do the symptoms of ADHD look like in girls?

Girls with ADHD tend to have more problems with inattention than hyperactivity. They also tend to be less disruptive than boys with ADHD. In girls, this inattention may appear as daydreaming, difficulty processing information or following directions, being distracted, "spacey" or "in her own world." Even when a girl is hyperactive, her behaviors may often look very different than they do in a boy. A girl with ADHD may be **hypertalkative** or **hyperreactive** (crying a lot or slamming doors)—behaviors one may not typically think of as being associated with ADHD. In addition to these behaviors, **Table 1** presents a summary of the

Girls with ADHD tend to have more problems with inattention than hyperactivity.

Table 1   Symptom Profile of Girls with ADHD

Acts before thinking	Difficulty remaining seated
Difficulty waiting for turn	Does not listen
Blunt answers	Loses things
Interrupts	Easily distracted
Talks excessively	Difficulty following instructions
Difficulty playing quietly	Difficulty sustaining attention
Fidgety	Shifts activities

Source: Biederman, J., Faraone, S. V., Mick, E., Williamson, S., Wilens, T.E., Spencer, T.J., et al. (1999). Clinical correlates of AD/HD in females: Findings from a large group of girls ascertained from pediatric and psychiatric referral sources. *Journal of the American Academy of Child and Adolescent Psychiatry, 38,* 966–975.

symptom profile of girls with ADHD as noted by Bei-
derman and colleagues in their study of girls with the
disorder (Biederman et al., 1999).

As a result of her ADHD symptoms, a girl may also
demonstrate a whole host of other behaviors. She may
react to distress experienced in the classroom (low self-
esteem and poor academic performance) by developing
avoidance behaviors exhibited by headaches or stomachaches or a true **school phobia** where she is unable
(or refuses) to attend school. She may become shy and
withdraw within the classroom (not answering questions or participating in class discussions). Poor organizational skills may occur in the form of messiness,
disheveled appearance, and/or grooming problems.
Her poor social skills exhibited by bossiness, shyness,
interrupting, or excessive talkativeness may result in
outright peer rejection or difficulty making and keeping
friends.

Adolescent females with ADHD have been found to
have more psychological distress than males with
ADHD. When compared to boys, girls with ADHD
report more anxiety, more distress, more depressive
symptoms, and feeling that they have no control over
what is going on in their lives (**external locus of control**)
(Rucklidge & Tannock, 2001). Because of these symptoms, girls with ADHD may be diagnosed correctly or
incorrectly as depressed, and their ADHD may be
missed. While their depressive symptoms may initially
respond to appropriate medications and therapy, these
girls will continue to struggle if their ADHD symptoms
are not diagnosed and treated as well.

6. *Are differences seen in women who have their ADHD diagnosed early versus later in life?*

To answer this question let's look at a study of women diagnosed with ADHD between 26 and 59 years of age. In general, these women were more apt to report a sense of things being beyond their control and a **learned helplessness** than women without ADHD. They also experienced more stress, anxiety, low self-esteem, and tended to give up easily when faced with difficult situations. In addition, they blamed themselves for their failures. This thinking often led to a vicious cycle, with women with ADHD being less likely to make an effort to finish tasks, which reinforced their sense of failure and inability to accomplish their goals, which only further increased their anxiety and depression. Women with ADHD were more likely than women without ADHD to have experienced depression, to have sought professional mental health treatment, and to have a greater use of medications to treat mental health conditions. In addition, they engaged in more emotion-oriented versus task oriented coping strategies than women without ADHD. They blamed themselves for not knowing what to do or how to act, and they were less likely to use effective problem-solving strategies (Rucklidge & Kaplan, 1997).

This study was also extremely valuable in pointing out that the diagnosis of ADHD helped these women feel more in control and more forgiving of their past mistakes. Putting a label on what they were experiencing provided a sense of relief for most women with ADHD. Early detection, especially in females, not only provides a sense of relief, but can also release them from the self-blame that accompanies the disorder prior to diagnosis. In other studies, women identified with ADHD in adulthood were found to not only have a greater degree of psychological distress, but also to have more frequent alcohol and drug use than males with ADHD. In addition, it was found that these addictive behaviors often began at an earlier age and were more severe than in males with the disorder (Wilens, Spencer, & Biederman, 1995).

7. Are certain subtypes of ADHD more common in females?

Over the years, females have been reported to have fewer hyperactive/impulsive and more inattentive symptoms and are diagnosed more frequently with ADHD-inattentive subtype. However, while the inattentive subtype of the disorder is most commonly seen in girls, results from recent clinical trials demonstrate that women with ADHD have a different presentation than that typically seen in girls. In a study of 536 adults with ADHD that included 188 women, 24% of these women were classified with inattentive subtype while 75% were diagnosed with combined subtype of the disorder (Robison et al., 2008). In men, 64% were diagnosed with combined subtype and 35% with inattentive subtype. The pure hyperactive/impulsive subtype was rarely seen in either men (3%) or women (1%).

8. Why is there an underdiagnosis of ADHD in girls and women compared to boys and men?

Despite the many studies that document ADHD exists in girls and that these girls tend to cluster more in the inattentive subtype, there has been little attention given to the finding that these girls are diagnosed less frequently than their male counterparts. Recently, however, a few experts have begun to look into the underdiagnosis of ADHD in girls, and we now have some clues as to the cause.

First, most standardized teacher and parent **rating scales** used for referral and aiding in the diagnosis of ADHD continue to emphasize externalizing symptoms such as hyperactivity and impulsivity. One study, designed to determine how mothers rated items on typical ADHD questionnaires, confirmed that mothers felt most items on standard ADHD rating scales more accurately described boys than girls. In addition, girls who were overlooked by their teachers and were seen by their parents as having ADHD characteristics, has led experts to conclude that parents may have been comparing their daughters to other girls, while teachers were comparing these same girls to their male classmates with ADHD. By comparing girls to their male counterparts, teachers may tend to dismiss the less obvious signs of ADHD in girls and not refer them for services (Ohan & Johnson, 2005).

These conclusions were confirmed in a study published in 2009, that explored disruptiveness as a factor for the gender gap in referrals of females. Findings in this study indicate that teachers referred girls with ADHD alone far less than girls with ADHD and oppositional defiant disorder or boys with ADHD (Ohan & Visser, 2009).

A further understanding of the differences in referrals for girls with ADHD, may be gained by looking at results from a **national survey** of 1797 adults (general public), 541 parents of children with ADHD, 550 teachers, and 346 children ages 12 to 17 years with ADHD conducted in 2004. Most of the public (58%) and the majority of teachers (82%) thought ADHD

Mothers felt most items on standard ADHD rating scales more accurately described boys than girls.

was more prevalent in boys. They similarly thought that boys were more likely to exhibit behavior problems than girls, while it was felt that girls were inattentive and depressed. Four out of ten teachers reported more difficulty in recognizing ADHD symptoms in girls and an overwhelming majority (85%) thought girls were more likely to go undiagnosed, thus confirming the reality of the situation. This overwhelming lack of information and a clear referral bias found in parents and teachers seem to be the main stumbling blocks to diagnosing girls and women and will need to be addressed if the problem of underdiagnosis is ever going to change.

Four out of ten teachers reported more difficulty in recognizing ADHD symptoms in girls.

9. How can this underdiagnosis of ADHD in females be addressed?

To tackle the underdiagnosis of ADHD in females, the problem must be attacked on several fronts. I have discussed the increased need for recognition of the disorder by teachers and parents in the answers to Questions 8 and 91, but clinicians also need to become more aware of the various presentations of this disorder as they vary by gender and by age. More specifically, clinicians need a set of revised criteria and guidelines that will lead to a more comprehensive and accurate diagnosis. Experts have come a long way in the last decade toward a better understanding of the way symptoms of ADHD differ in men and women, but there is still much work to be done. To properly diagnos ADHD, especially in women, we need to look at the whole picture. In addition, clinicians need a new set of criteria that are more relevant and developmentally appropriate for adults. The APA is currently evaluating criteria for the diagnosis of ADHD and proposing several changes in DSM-5, in particular, the age of onset criterion that states that symptoms must be present by the age of 7 to make a diagnosis of ADHD. (If you are interested in other changes being proposed, see Appendix A for a more in-depth discussion of this topic.) Let's take a look at some of the other aspects of ADHD that may change over time, resulting in an underdiagnosis in females.

Parents, teachers, and clinicians alike also need to become aware that developmentally, there appears to be a significant shift in ADHD symptoms with age. While the symptom of inattentiveness seems to be fairly stable over time (63% of girls with inattentive subtype retained that diagnosis at follow-up); and hyperactivity, which may be prominent in younger children, decreases with age. In 2006, Dr. Stephen Hinshaw and his colleagues reported a follow-up study of adolescent girls with ADHD they conducted. In that study, almost two-thirds of the girls who had previously been diagnosed as having combined subtype in childhood either met criteria for the inattentive subtype (23.5%) or no longer met criteria for the diagnosis of ADHD (34%) at follow-up as symptoms of the hyperactive/impulsive subtype decreased or disappeared altogether (Hinshaw et al., 2006). Unfortunately, these changes in diagnosis did not mean that girls no longer have symptoms or day-to-day problems. Instead, they did not exhibit enough symptoms to meet criteria for the diagnosis as it must currently be defined. The same situation may also be true for women with inattention persisting and predominating into adulthood. As inattention is more difficult to diagnose than hyperactivity, this shift in symptoms may result in ADHD being overlooked in these females.

In addition, it seems that over time, deficiencies in executive functioning (e.g., organization and time-management skills) become a more prominent feature of ADHD as expectations increase for women during adulthood. To clarify the picture of ADHD and for a more accurate diagnosis in women, therefore, the focus

Over time, deficiencies in executive functioning (e.g., organization and time-management skills) become a more prominent feature of ADHD as expectations increase for women during adulthood.

needs to shift from behavior issues (hyperactivity and oppositional behaviors) seen in childhood to symptoms that reflect the reported executive functioning difficulties in organization and problem solving that plague older teens and adults with ADHD. Complaints from women with ADHD mainly center on the degree of difficulty they have completing tasks that other women seem to be able to accomplish with little effort, and their sense of being overwhelmed by everyday activities. Women spend countless hours trying to cope at work and at home, with no clue that the difficulties they encounter are the result of a real disorder that can be effectively managed and treated once the diagnosis is made.

10. Does a high IQ and hard work lessen the impact of the symptoms of ADHD and delay the diagnosis in girls and women?

The diagnosis of ADHD has been reported to be delayed if a person has protective influences such as a high **IQ (intelligence quotient)**, a supportive family, relatively good social skills, and no serious behavior problems (Tzelepis, Schubiner, & Warbasse, 1995). Girls with ADHD and superior IQs may be able to compensate academically for many years. By not calling attention to themselves behaviorally, socially, or academically, they run the risk of not being diagnosed until later in life, if at all. In one study, Yale psychologists Thomas E. Brown and Donald Quinlan evaluated 74 students, aged 7 to 18 years, with IQ scores above 120 (in the top 9% of the population), referred for chronic underachievement. Most of these students had no behavioral problems and were not hyperactive, but they did have attention deficits. Students in this study had experienced 2 to 10 years of deteriorating grades before their attention problems were recognized. After only 3 months of treatment

Girls with ADHD and superior IQs may be able to compensate academically for many years.

with appropriate medication for their ADHD, 81% of these students had improved significantly in their academic work (Brown, 1998).

Delays in diagnosis and treatment are often seen in females because girls work harder to compensate or hide their symptoms in an effort to meet parent and/or teacher expectations. Therefore, they may not demonstrate academic difficulties or have problems in the classroom during their early years. As time progresses and demands increase, however, it becomes increasingly difficult for females with ADHD to compensate, particularly in college or in graduate or professional level academic settings. Whether a disorder can be considered to exist if one is able to compensate for it remains an issue of controversy. However, what remains true is that many females with ADHD are able to perform well academically during early school years because of hard work and various coping strategies. These same girls often demonstrate significant symptoms of ADHD and depression as demands increase in middle school, high school, and beyond. Therefore, the take-home message for parents, teachers, and clinicians is this: Good grades and satisfactory teacher reports cannot be used to rule out ADHD in girls.

Girls work harder to compensate or hide their symptoms in an effort to meet parent and/or teacher expectations.

The diagnosis of ADHD in these bright girls who have done well academically and who may not exhibit typical symptoms is often a challenge. For parents, the following list of questions about your daughter's behavior may help you to determine if she is having significant difficulties despite her high IQ:

Good grades and satisfactory teacher reports cannot be used to rule out ADHD in girls.

1. Does she have a poor sense of time?
2. Does she struggle with procrastination, typically beginning homework when it is nearly time for bed?

3. Is she a night owl who seems to get a second wind later in the evening?

4. Is she an "absentminded professor?"

5. Does she hyperfocus to the extent that she does not hear you when you call?

6. Is she a dawdler who has great difficulty getting up on time in the morning and getting ready for school once she is out of bed?

7. Is she very likely to misplace personal items—jackets, keys, wallets, and so forth?

8. Do you find that you need to repeat multistep directions because she has not been able to register all of the steps?

9. Do you send her upstairs for something only to find that she completely forgets her mission and is sidetracked by something else?

(Adapted from Nadeau, K., 2004. *Does your gifted child have AD/HD?* Retrieved from http://www.addvance.com/help/parents/gifted_child.html.)

The girl whose parents answer "yes" to many, if not all, of these questions presents a very different picture from the typical child with ADHD, who is impulsive, **overactive**, and with little inclination to follow the rules. Yet, she may be just as affected by her inattention, distractibility, and poor executive skills as her hyperactive counterparts.

Julia speaks:

These questions describe my now 18-year-old daughter to perfection from the time she was in elementary school. Yet, she made almost perfect grades all the way through high school, so I never thought ADHD was a possibility, even though she herself said that she thought she had ADHD.

I blew it off because of her school performance and because I had a picture in my head of a stereotypical, hyperactive child as being one with ADHD. Not my smart little girl, who was shy and not a behavior problem. But, oh, how I wish I had paid more attention and done my research. If I had realized these were ADHD characteristics, maybe she wouldn't have developed depression, anxiety, and a very entrenched eating disorder. I can't believe I missed her ADHD for so many years!

11. Are societal stereotypes and ignorance harming a lot of women and young girls with ADHD and causing them to slip through the cracks?

For a woman or girl with ADHD, her most painful challenge is often the struggle she has with her own overwhelming sense of inadequacy in fulfilling the roles that she feels are expected of her by her family and by society. Girls are raised to internalize—to take in and own negative feedback, to apologize, to accommodate, and to not stand up for themselves. Boys, however, are typically raised to externalize—to fight when attacked, and to place blame for the problem outside of themselves. For example, if a boy fails an exam, he dismisses the matter by saying it was a "stupid test." However, if a girl fails the same test, she responds with the overwhelming sense that she is stupid. These differences are described very tellingly in Sari Solden's book, *Women With Attention Deficit Disorder*, in which she writes of "coming out of the ADD closet" of shame and self-blame.

Trying to live up to traditional **gender-role expectations** can take a great toll on the psychological well-being of women with ADHD. In one study, when women with a

Trying to live up to traditional gender-role expectations can take a great toll on the psychological well-being of women with ADHD.

diagnosis of ADHD were compared to women who did not have ADHD or any other psychiatric diagnoses, the women with ADHD rated themselves significantly different from their perception of the ideal woman than did the women without ADHD. Women with ADHD compared themselves less favorably to most women on 12 positive traits, namely—being assertive, loving, active, successful at work, self-confident, logical, romantic, independent, intelligent, self-disciplined, rational, and having leadership ability—than did women without ADHD. Women with ADHD were reported to have a significantly lower level sense of well-being in the areas of self-acceptance, control over their environment, positive relations with others, autonomy, and purpose in life, but not in personal growth (Burton, 2005). Overall, these findings confirm the psychological suffering that women with ADHD experience and the overall loss of their sense of well-being, as they struggle to meet gender-role norms and deal with their ADHD on a daily basis.

Without the benefit of a diagnosis, girls and women with ADHD are often not only at the mercy of their own self-blame, but are also subjected to the misunderstanding and stereotyping of society in general. I vividly recall receiving an e-mail from a woman who was newly diagnosed with ADHD. She shared her relief at the diagnosis and marveled at her excellent response to medication, and then went on to state that she had recently dyed her hair red. At that point, I mused that perhaps her impulsivity was not under as good control as she had thought. However, upon continued reading of the e-mail, I found that she had added, "I'm tired of being referred to as a *dumb blonde!*"

The burden of undiagnosed ADHD is also experienced differently by girls than boys with ADHD. When compared to boys, girls reported more often that it was "very difficult" for them to get things done, to focus on schoolwork, to get along with parents, and to make friends. Girls with ADHD are also more likely to feel embarrassed by their ADHD symptoms, resulting in reactive behaviors of acting out or withdrawal. With a broader awareness of ADHD and better understanding of the differences in its presentation in girls and boys, it is hoped that girls will no longer have to suffer silently with the many burdens that the disorder presents for them.

Girls with ADHD are also more likely to feel embarrassed by their ADHD symptoms.

12. Do girls who are diagnosed in childhood fare better as they enter adolescence?

To answer this question, let's examine a 5-year follow-up study that takes a look at girls who were diagnosed with ADHD during their elementary school years and compares them to non-ADHD girls (Hinshaw et. al., 2006). This groundbreaking study contained several key findings that deserve discussion. Primarily, this study presented overwhelming evidence that girls diagnosed during elementary school did not outgrow ADHD, with the majority continuing to demonstrate significant impairments in functioning 5 years later. According to study results, only 16% of girls diagnosed with ADHD were considered to be well-adjusted in adolescence compared to 86% of girls without ADHD.

In addition, these girls with ADHD were found to have continuing impairments despite the fact that 70% received some form of therapy and 80% accessed school-based services during the intervening years.

Why would this be the case? Additional study findings may hold a clue. When the results were analyzed, only 24% of the girls with inattentive subtype and only 45% of the combined subtype were still on stimulant medication! I personally feel that this failure to continue medication treatment for ADHD may be the reason why so few of these girls who were diagnosed in childhood were showing a positive adjustment in adolescence, despite the fact that girls and their families had accessed some other form of therapy. If that is the case, the next question should be, why were so few of these girls receiving medications to treat their ADHD, when the symptoms were clearly continuing to cause impairments?

Parents, physicians, and mental health professionals may be unaware of the fact that ADHD is a chronic condition.

The answer to this question was not found in this study; however, several possibilities come to mind. First, parents, physicians, and mental health professionals may be unaware of the fact that ADHD is a chronic condition with symptoms continuing into adolescence and adulthood. Second, girls or their parents may discontinue therapy either because they are unaware that the initial improvement of ADHD symptoms is *not* a cure and that symptoms will return quickly when medication is withdrawn; or they discontinue therapy because they experience side effects. Third, other symptoms may have developed that overshadowed the ADHD. We know that girls with ADHD suffer silently and exhibit more depression and anxiety as they enter adolescence. If this occurs, they would then focus on and seek treatment for those symptoms, forgetting that the ADHD is still there. Or perhaps, these girls and their families may have just given up and become resigned to the inability to function on the same level as other girls without ADHD.

In this study, girls with the inattentive subtype ADHD were found to be just as severely affected at follow-up as girls with the combined-subtype ADHD. This finding is extremely important as many parents and professionals often think that the inattentive subtype ADHD, because hyperactivity is absent, is a milder form of ADHD or is somehow of less consequence for these girls. In actuality, the opposite may be the case.

It should also be noted that in this study the mere perception of academic competence was often associated with more positive adolescent outcomes. Girls with ADHD who were more confident about their ability to succeed academically in elementary school showed reduced levels of mood disorders and acting out behaviors, actual gains in academic achievement, and lower levels of substance abuse in adolescence. Thus, self-perceived academic competence, regardless of actual academic achievement, may help protect girls from negative outcomes resulting from their ADHD symptoms.

Brenda speaks:

My 13-year-old daughter was diagnosed with ADD in 4th grade. When she started taking stimulant medication there was a marked difference in her academic achievement as well as her demeanor. She became less argumentative and basically a happier person. We tried not medicating her on the weekends, but she was so argumentative and unfocused that we even started medicating her on the weekends. She entered puberty a couple of months ago. Her schoolwork has started to slip (forgetting assignments, poor test grades, etc.) and for several months she has been running her fingers through the bottom of her long hair—it seems to be something she does not even realize she is doing.

Girls with the inattentive subtype ADHD were found to be just as severely affected at follow-up as girls with the combined-subtype ADHD.

ADHD in Women and Girls: What Are the Differences?

Yesterday, we took her for her ADD checkup and told the doctor all of this. He said that many times when children enter puberty their ADD symptoms decrease or stop entirely and that playing with her hair was a sign that she did not need the medication anymore. Frankly, we went with the intention of asking to increase/change/add to her medication as we have seen symptoms worsening. He attributed the increase in argumentative behavior as normal teenage rebellion. He suggested that we take her off medication and see what happens. Everything I have read states that boys' symptoms may decrease with puberty, but that girls' symptoms tend to increase, and possibly the first symptoms of hyperactivity would appear in girls during this stage (playing with hair). I feel the doctor is wrong, but don't know what to do at this point! This is all very confusing! My daughter's ADD seems worse now that she is an adolescent.

13. What are the risks in adolescence for girls with ADHD?

As discussed in the answer to Question 12, few girls diagnosed with ADHD in childhood show positive adjustment during adolescence, with only 16% of girls doing well overall. Over the years, these girls have been found to be at greater risk for many problem behaviors including sexual acting out, substance abuse, cigarette smoking, and eating disorders. Teachers have confirmed these findings, reporting that they have observed gender differences in the risky behaviors associated with ADHD. For example, more teachers reported promiscuous behavior to be more common in girls (44%) than boys (28%) with ADHD (Quinn & Wigal, 2004). These problems exhibited by girls with ADHD were not found to be isolated to impulsive acting out, either.

Accumulating evidence also suggests that girls with the inattentive subtype of ADHD were less likely to show an overall positive adjustment at follow-up than girls diagnosed with ADHD combined subtype. As a result of their ADHD symptoms and negative experiences, all girls with ADHD are more likely to make poor decisions and to have poor problem-solving skills. They often blame themselves as they have no other explanation as to why they struggle in school and at home. To ease their pain or to self-medicate, these girls may turn to drugs, alcohol, or food. Over the years, I have seen many girls with anxiety and feelings of helplessness try to control their lives by controlling their eating, resulting in anorexia and/or other disordered eating patterns.

Rayette speaks:

My daughter, who is now 30, and I have both been diagnosed with ADHD. Now being 50, I look back on my life, especially my childhood and realize that most of my complications and setbacks were a result of having ADHD and not being diagnosed at an early age. My daughter was diagnosed at a young age, but has suffered immensely from ADHD to the degree that she became an addict, self-medicating in her adolescent years to help her live adequately from her point of view) in society. She is now in recovery and doing quite well. I wish I had known about the risks that she faced as an adolescent girl with ADHD; I might have been able to get help for her sooner.

14. Does ADHD affect self-esteem in girls and women?

Girls and women with ADHD often feel that they are not good at anything and that things are not going to change for them anytime soon. Unfortunately, the

Girls and women with ADHD often feel that they are not good at anything.

damage done to a girl's **self-esteem**, when she has ADHD, comes all too early as she struggles to keep up appearances in school and at home while at the same time dealing with the disapproval of her parents, teachers, and others. Comparing herself to other girls, a girl with ADHD quickly becomes convinced that she is different. For those girls with combined subtype ADHD, society only adds to this perception with its criticism of hyperactive, messy, disorganized, or typical tomboy behaviors. There is no excuse such as "boys will be boys" for girls with ADHD!

Comparing herself to other girls, a girl with ADHD quickly becomes convinced that she is different.

There is no excuse such as "boys will be boys" for girls with ADHD!

Research has confirmed that these negative self-perceptions and has also highlighted the fact that women with ADHD struggle with a more negative self-image than do men with ADHD (Arcia & Conners, 1998). For most of her life, a woman with ADHD has experienced a negative image of herself, whether it was maternal disapproval and teacher criticism that she endured as a young girl, or society's criticism of her impulsive, risk-taking behaviors during her teen years. These long-held negative feelings and self-criticism, rather than the cognitive challenges of ADHD, are most likely the cause of most of the psychological damage and mental health issues seen in women with ADHD (Rucklidge & Kaplan, 1997).

Early detection of ADHD is critical to preventing poor self-esteem.

Early detection of ADHD is, therefore, critical to preventing poor self-esteem, especially if girls and women are to free themselves from self-blame and the feeling that everything is their fault. Without a diagnostic label to help them interpret the problems and academic struggles they experienced in childhood and during postsecondary school, these women often see themselves as defective and not very smart. When I diagnose a woman with ADHD, her first response is often, "Is that all it is? I thought I was stupid!" Challenging this pattern of thinking is the crucial first step to maintaining self-esteem, preventing depression and other mental health issues, and dispelling the myths associated with ADHD in women and girls with ADHD.

15. If ADHD is a chronic lifelong disorder, can I expect to experience similar issues and problems for the rest of my life?

ADHD is indeed a lifelong condition with symptoms persisting well into adulthood for the majority of individuals with the disorder. However, the impact of these symptoms may vary depending on the environment and a host of other circumstances that a woman finds herself in. When researchers followed children who had been diagnosed with ADHD in elementary school, they found that approximately 65% continued to have symptoms that affected their functioning as adults. The good news is that almost half of adults, despite the fact that they still might have had symptoms, were not impaired! So, while your symptoms many continue, you need not feel that you are condemned to suffer for the rest of your life. The next question that needs to be investigated, however, is what can *you* do to ensure that you are in the group of women with ADHD who are doing well?

ADHD is a lifelong condition with symptoms persisting well into adulthood for the majority of individuals with the disorder.

Improving Your Outcome

Once you are aware of your ADHD diagnosis, there are several steps you can take to increase your chance of gaining control of your symptoms and your life. You know your needs better than anyone and are your own best advocate. Read, ask questions, and gather as much information as possible. Schedule a comprehensive evaluation to not only provide a formal diagnosis, but to also delineate a clear picture of your strengths and weaknesses. You will then be ready to participate in designing a total treatment plan that meets your unique needs.

Get Treatment

An effective, total treatment program is essential to future success.

An effective, **total treatment program** is essential to future success. Such programs usually include a combination of medication, **psychotherapy**, coaching, alternative treatments, and necessary related services (support groups, counseling, family therapy, etc.). ADHD can have serious consequences, but it is treatable with safe and effective medications that can change people's lives. (See Question 35 for a more in-depth discussion of medications used to treat ADHD.)

Deal with Coexisting Conditions

A comprehensive evaluation will not only confirm your ADHD and outline your strengths and weaknesses, but also identify any related or coexisting conditions. For optimum functioning, these conditions will need to be diagnosed and possibly treated in addition to your ADHD. Depression, **addiction**, and poor social skills can all impact your day-to-day functioning and will need to be addressed.

Make ADHD-Friendly Life Choices

What else can you do to ensure success? First, simplify your life and avoid or reduce stress wherever and whenever you can. Then, make sure that the choices you make are as ADHD-friendly as possible, allowing you to use your strengths rather than continually wrestling with weaknesses caused by your ADHD symptoms. Pursuing a healthy lifestyle (exercising, getting enough sleep, and eating properly) will also help you feel and function better.

Develop Necessary Skills

Any skill deficits will also need to be addressed. These include time-management, organization, and communication skills. Mastering work-related skills and choosing an ADHD-friendly career (see Question 66 for a further explanation of what this entails) will provide both job satisfaction and economic stability.

16. Is ADHD genetically inherited?

ADHD is primarily an inherited disorder. It is estimated that genetic predisposition is a contributing factor in 60% to 80% of ADHD cases. For the remainder, ADHD may be the result of environmental exposure or early brain injury that impedes normal brain development. Exposure to chronic low levels of lead, pesticides, prematurity, maternal obstetrical complications during the pregnancy, exposure to cigarette smoke before birth, malnourishment, and other illnesses, such as meningitis or encephalitis, in infants and toddlers can all result in learning and attention problems.

ADHD is primarily an inherited disorder.

To date, researchers have identified hundreds of gene variations that occur more frequently in children with ADHD than those without ADHD. Many of these genes have long been known to be important in learning, attention, and behaviors. In ADHD, parts of these genes have been found to be missing or to have extra repeated stretches of DNA in areas that affect brain functioning. There are hundreds of such genes that can be affected in each person. Yet, despite these numerous genetic variations, each person ends up with a similar result—ADHD. These variations, however, may be an explanation for why people with ADHD all have such different symptom presentations.

ADHD in Women and Girls: What Are the Differences?

Currently, there is no commonly available genetic test for ADHD.

Currently, there is no commonly available **genetic test** for ADHD. Research continues to focus on identifying which genes, or combination of genes, may cause a person to be more susceptible to ADHD. Until that time, the diagnosis of ADHD is made by compiling a list of symptoms and looking at past history and a family history during a comprehensive clinical interview. An in-depth family history is often very revealing. **Family trees** can be created to help identify those family members who display symptoms of ADHD, including those adults who were never diagnosed. Despite the lack of a formal diagnosis, discussing your family history with your doctor may reveal characteristics that doctors commonly see in adults with ADHD, such as an inability to settle down, dropping out of high school or college, changing jobs frequently, having difficulty completing projects, organizing their lives or having multiple relationships or marriages.

PART TWO

ADHD and Coexisting Conditions Commonly Seen in Women and Girls

Girls with ADHD are often anxious. Is this anxiety secondary to ADHD or a separate condition?

Can significant traumas early in life precipitate ADHD?

Can a person with ADHD also have a learning disability?

More . . .

17. Is ADHD usually seen alone, or do other conditions accompany the diagnosis, and are they specific to gender?

It is estimated that 70% to 75% of adults seeking treatment for ADHD have at least one additional psychiatric diagnosis.

It is estimated that 70% to 75% of adults seeking treatment for ADHD have at least one additional psychiatric diagnosis. While there is general agreement that gender-related differences exist in these coexisting conditions, these differences have usually been described in clusters—where boys have been found to have more externalizing disruptive behavior disorders and girls have been described as tending to have more internalizing disorders such as anxiety and depression. While research in women continues to lag behind that looking at adult males with ADHD, many clinicians are reporting unique issues and coexisting conditions in women with ADHD within their practices. In a 1995 study by Stein and colleagues, women with ADHD commonly reported dysphoria or chronic low-level irritability and depressed mood, along with problems with attention and organization, conduct, and impulsivity. Men, however, were more likely to report conduct and learning problems, stress intolerance, attention difficulties, poor social skills, and awkwardness.

18. Are the other conditions that frequently accompany ADHD evident in childhood, or do they develop later due to environmental influences?

Coexisting conditions appear early on in the picture of ADHD, but how early is the critical question. In one study comparing 165 four- to six-year-olds to 381 seven- to nine-year-olds, similar rates of impairment were found in school, social, and overall functioning. We can also look at a more recent study designed to assess the effectiveness and safety of the stimulant, methylphenidate, for the treatment of ADHD in **preschoolers** to determine what coexisting conditions can be found at this early age. In this study, 8% of the preschoolers were reported to have an anxiety disorder, 52% had oppositional defiant disorder, and 2% had **conduct disorder**. Seventy-six percent of this sample were male and all had combined or hyperactive/impulsive subtype ADHD, which probably accounts for the high percentage of externalizing behavior disorders (Greenhill et al., 2006).

Oppositional defiant disorder (ODD) is seen about half as frequently in girls with ADHD as boys with ADHD. In studies of elementary school-aged populations, girls were noted to have more anxiety and mood disorders than behavior disorders. Low self-esteem and shame developed over time in these girls with ADHD, but many women tell me that they had experienced embarrassment from their symptoms early on (some as early as 8 years of age). Elementary school-aged girls with ADHD who do well academically have often already paid a high price in terms of their self-worth. Their need to work hard and put in more time to perform simple tasks is often translated (by themselves and others) into not being as smart as other children in whom learning goes more smoothly. In one study by Joseph Biederman and his coinvestigators, published in *Biological Psychiatry* in 2006, girls diagnosed with ADHD in childhood were seen to have a greater incidence of psychotic mood or anxiety disorders as they entered their 20s. Rates of these disorders increased over time, with up to about 60% exhibiting one of these problems compared to control subjects (25%) in young adulthood, but the roots can be found in early childhood.

Oppositional defiant disorder is seen about half as frequently in girls with ADHD as boys with ADHD.

19. When a diagnosis of ADHD is not made until well into adulthood, do women with ADHD develop addictions?

The **ADHD–addiction** connection is a significant problem for women and girls with ADHD and is often an attempt to self-medicate their undiagnosed and, therefore, untreated ADHD symptoms. Shame, self-blame, and isolation often contribute to the pain and suffering caused by ADHD symptoms, leading these women to abuse substances such as drugs and alcohol. In addition to **substance abuse**, cigarette smoking, compulsive shopping, and out-of-control spending have all been reported in women with ADHD. Studies confirm that girls with ADHD begin smoking cigarettes early in life, and that they smoke more cigarettes per day than boys. In addition to cigarette smoking, adolescents and adults with ADHD develop more severe and chronic substance use disorders. Other conditions such as anxiety, depression, and bipolar disorder often seen along with ADHD, particularly in females, may also increase the risk of substance abuse and addictive behaviors.

Studies confirm that girls with ADHD begin smoking cigarettes early in life, and that they smoke more cigarettes per day than boys.

Women and teenage girls with ADHD may experience problems with finances as they spend more than they can afford, using credit cards to soothe away the day-to-day fallout of their disorder. Shopping can be used as a way to deal with depression or anxiety or to create excitement or stimulation. Women with ADHD may be particularly vulnerable to compulsive shopping because their impulsivity makes it hard for them to think through the purchase, and they often buy items that they do not need. These women shop to make themselves feel better. They go shopping with the intention of buying one or two items and return with bags full of purchases, resulting over time in serious financial difficulties. This impulsivity may also be seen with credit card purchases. I have worked with many female college students, who having received several new credit cards cannot resist the urge to spend to the limit of each, only to graduate with a significant credit card debt hanging over their heads.

Regardless of the addiction, recovery for many of these women may present a significant challenge. According to Wendy Richardson, author of *The Link Between ADD and Addictions* (1997) and *When Too Much Isn't Enough* (2005), women with ADHD are often unaware that their undiagnosed ADHD is a large part of the complex set of problems with which they are struggling. She further cautions that recovery from addictions can be difficult, if not impossible, for these women without proper diagnosis and treatment. However, many of these women, when diagnosed, are faced with the additional challenge of convincing their physician that they are not automatically at risk for abusing their stimulant medication. In fact, just the opposite appears to be true. Women are at a low risk of abusing their ADHD medication when involved in a comprehensive treatment program. In fact, treatment for ADHD allows these women to stay in recovery, whether from abuse of drugs, alcohol, money, or food.

Regardless of the addiction, recovery for many of these women may present a significant challenge.

20. How frequently are depression and other mood disorders seen in women and girls with ADHD?

For some time, it has been known that women with ADHD are more likely to **internalize symptoms** and become anxious, depressed, and to suffer **emotional dysregulation** than males with the disorder. Recent evidence confirms that girls with ADHD are more likely to be diagnosed with **major depression** and to be treated for depression prior to their ADHD diagnosis. Findings from the preliminary analysis of a comorbidity study involving 3559 individuals with ADHD, ranging in age from 2 to 88 years, confirmed an increase in mood disorders in females (Turgay et al., 2006). In studies, women with ADHD were found to report higher rates than men for major depression, anxiety disorders, and dysthymic disorders. However, the greatest increased risk was for the co-occurrence of major depression. Girls with ADHD were found to be 5.4 times more likely to be diagnosed with major depression than girls without the condition. In addition, major depression in girls with ADHD had an earlier onset; lasted more than twice as long (3 years in girls with ADHD compared to 1.3 years in girls without ADHD); was associated with greater impairment, such as thoughts of suicide; and required more intensive treatment, including psychiatric hospitalization.

Girls with ADHD were found to be 5.4 times more likely to be diagnosed with major depression than girls without the condition.

21. Is depression diagnosed more commonly before or after ADHD?

As we have seen, ADHD often leads to **demoralization** and chronic low-grade depression (**dysthymia**). In many females with ADHD, the depressive symptoms that accompany ADHD have the potential to overshadow, complicate, or delay the ADHD diagnosis altogether. Because of these secondary symptoms, girls and women with ADHD are frequently diagnosed, correctly or incorrectly, as depressed, and the ADHD as the primary or coexisting diagnosis may be missed. While symptoms specific to these coexisting disorders may respond to appropriate antidepressant medication and therapy, these girls continue to struggle if their ADHD symptoms are not also treated.

The depressive symptoms that accompany ADHD have the potential to overshadow, complicate, or delay the ADHD diagnosis.

When depressive symptoms predominate, adolescent girls with ADHD are more likely to be treated for depression rather than their ADHD symptoms. In a nationwide survey conducted in April 2002, by Harris Interactive, 14% of girls (ages 13 to 17) with ADHD were found to have been treated with antidepressants prior to their ADHD diagnosis compared to only 5% of males with ADHD. Fifty-six percent of these girls also reported that they felt better knowing the name of their disorder once their ADHD was diagnosed (Quinn & Wigal, 2004). When the ADHD is finally diagnosed and treated with appropriate doses of stimulant medication, the depressive symptoms often recede, as they were the result of untreated ADHD and not a primary coexisting condition.

Amy speaks:

It would be a good idea for therapists to do an ADHD evaluation on all women who complain about anxiety/depression. I've been to five or six therapists over the years—diagnosis: depression. Not one ever even suggested I might have the ADHD. My boss, a school principal, was the first one to suggest that to me. I was not diagnosed by a psychiatrist until I was 63, but too much damage has been done. I'm a teacher who has lost many jobs. My finances have always been a mess. I've had to retire with no pension. I sure wish the diagnosis was made earlier!

22. Can ADHD be seen with bipolar disorder, or are women misdiagnosed as having bipolar disorder instead of ADHD?

Perhaps the most difficult diagnosis to make in women is that of ADHD-combined subtype and its accompanying demoralization versus **bipolar mood disorder (BMD)**, because these two disorders have so many features in common including mood fluctuations, increased energy levels, hypertalkativeness, impulsivity, racing thoughts, irritability, and problems with sleep. In addition, they both have a chronic course with lifelong impairment, as well as a strong genetic component.

ADHD is about 10 times more common than BMD, however. In adults, the two disorders can be seen together with the ADHD symptoms beginning in childhood. Recent studies estimate that 20% to 25% of adults with BMD also have ADHD, while only 6% to 7% of adults with ADHD have BMD. Several studies have demonstrated that the earlier that mood swings of bipolar disorder start, the more likely it is that a person has coexisting ADHD with 80% of children and one-third of adolescents diagnosed with BMD also having ADHD (Geller & Luby, 1997). Consequently, unless the person making the diagnosis is careful, there is a substantial risk of misdiagnosis or of a missed diagnosis. I have often seen ADHD misdiagnosed as BMD in women and girls when depression and combined type ADHD occurred together.

ADHD and BMD do have several differences that can be of help when trying to sort out the correct diagnosis.

ADHD and BMD do have several differences that can be of help when trying to sort out the correct diagnosis. These include a person's age when symptoms first occur; the persistence of symptoms; sleep patterns; the characteristics of the mood fluctuations including their duration, stability, and whether the mood fluctuations are in response to real stimuli in the environment; and family history. To help differentiate these two diagnoses, let's briefly take a look at each of these factors separately.

- **Age of onset**. ADHD symptoms are present throughout the life span. For a diagnosis to be made, symptoms must occur (although not necessarily impair functioning) by age 7. BMD can be seen in young children, but symptoms more commonly begin during adolescence or young adulthood. Therefore, symptoms that begin prior to puberty are usually ADHD.

- **Persistence of symptoms**. In addition to earlier onset, the symptoms of ADHD are always present, while the manic symptoms of BMD come and go with normal moods occurring between episodes. A woman with ADHD is *always* hypertalkative and impulsive, not just during manic or hypomanic states.

- **Sleep patterns**. Individuals with ADHD and those with BMD both have problems with sleep. However, with ADHD, a woman may chronically have difficulty falling asleep or awaken early, thus not be getting enough sleep, but she would like to get more. By contrast, someone with BMD may have a reduced need for sleep. During a manic phase, a woman can often function quite well with little or no sleep until she actually becomes psychotic.

- **Mood swings**. Women and girls with ADHD often have strong emotional reactions to the real events in their lives. Positive occurrences (a good test grade or a great shopping bargain) can result in excitement and a happy mood, but just as quickly, negative ones (a flat tire or not receiving an invitation to a party) can cause a bad mood. This clear triggering of mood shifts by real events characteristically distinguishes ADHD from bipolar mood shifts that come and go unrelated to life events often leaving a woman to wonder why she feels the way she does. In addition, because ADHD mood swings occur as a result of real events happening in the environment, these moods can shift rapidly, sometimes within minutes. Conversely, the mood swings of BMD often occur over days or weeks even in the most rapid cyclers. A **rapid-cycling bipolar disorder** is defined as one in which an individual experiences at least four shifts of mood over a year. Many women with ADHD have that many mood shifts in a single day!

- **Racing thoughts**. Women with BMD often report that they have racing thoughts, while those with ADHD describe their thoughts, usually while trying to fall asleep, as jumping around from one unrelated topic or worry to the next. Unfortunately, however, if a woman with ADHD describes her thoughts while falling asleep as racing, many physicians may incorrectly diagnosis her as having BMD.

- **Family history**. Both ADHD and BMD have a genetic component. Therefore, when taking a family history, it is important to seek out symptoms of both disorders, as they may not have been formally diagnosed in the past. As pointed out earlier, some women may have both ADHD and BMD and one or the other or both may also occur in their families. It is important that when ADHD and BMD occur together, both must be properly diagnosed *and* treated in order for these women to improve.

23. How are coexisting ADHD and bipolar disorder best treated?

When a woman has ADHD and BMD, both conditions must be treated in order for her to improve completely. In cases where only BMD is diagnosed and treated, and undiagnosed ADHD symptoms remain, a woman will be somewhat better but she will continue to exhibit impulsive/hyperactive symptoms, and it may look like her BMD is not responding to treatment. In such instances, many clinicians will prescribe additional medications to treat her bipolar disorder and the woman ends up on multiple medication combinations (and their accompanying side effects) while not really getting much better. For best results, it is imperative to treat both disorders. However, the BMD must be treated first before treatment of the ADHD symptoms in order to prevent making the situation worse.

Treatment of BMD is accomplished with a **mood stabilizer**. The mood stabilizer should be prescribed first and taken consistently (even when symptoms of the mood disorder have improved) to avoid the risk of triggering a **manic or depressive episode** when a stimulant is added to treat the ADHD symptoms. Once the BMD symptoms have been stabilized for a few weeks on medication and the symptoms are under control, a stimulant can be added to treat the ADHD without worrying about causing a manic episode or the return of any psychotic symptoms. As with the treatment of any patient with ADHD, the dose of stimulant medication should be adjusted slowly. Doses should start low and be increased in small increments every few days or weeks, until symptoms improve. Although treating ADHD and BMD is a complex undertaking, the majority of women with both conditions can live relatively stable lives if they work with a therapist skilled in treating both disorders.

Amy speaks:

I have ADHD, but have also recently been diagnosed with bipolar disorder, being treated with lithium and Prozac (fluoxetine). At first, I was not being treated for my ADHD from a medical/psychological standpoint and

I continued to have problems in this area. I had trouble with paying attention, making decisions, and completing my work. Once I sought additional psychiatric help and research to get a proper diagnosis and treatment, things really improved for me. I now feel that maybe I can live a productive life and accomplish the goals that I have set for myself. I want to go back to school and get a degree in design, as well as have a family These dreams all seemed impossible before I got diagnosed and treated for both conditions.

24. Girls with ADHD are often anxious. Is this anxiety secondary to ADHD or a separate condition?

In general, there are three scenarios to consider when it comes to ADHD and anxiety. First, a great many girls and women with ADHD commonly experience anxiety as a result of their untreated ADHD symptoms; second, in some females, ADHD can be accompanied by a separate and clinically significant anxiety disorder independent of their ADHD; and third, girls and women with an anxiety disorder may look like they have ADHD, but in reality, the poor attention and **concentration** difficulties they exhibit are directly the result of the anxiety disorder, not ADHD.

Deciding whether a girl has anxiety, ADHD, or both can often be challenging given the overlap in symptoms between these two disorders. When the two conditions are seen together, it may be impossible to answer the question of whether the anxiety symptoms are because of or in addition to the ADHD. Girls with ADHD often worry that their ADHD symptoms may cause them embarrassment or sabotage their efforts. Likewise, the preoccupying worry of a **generalized anxiety disorder** may limit a young girl's ability to pay attention, focus, and respond to daily demands. Physical symptoms such as fidgetiness, hair pulling, nail biting, or inability to sit still may be symptoms of both anxiety and ADHD. As stated earlier, many girls and women with ADHD develop anxiety as a result of the embarrassment and humiliation caused by their ADHD symptoms. They fear that their symptoms will sabotage them as they have in the past and become anxious that this will happen again. However, with a generalized anxiety disorder, girls and women are usually preoccupied with worry about real or imagined issues. This preoccupation may make it difficult for them to study or get work done. It may also limit school attendance. In girls and women with ADHD, anxiety is mainly around their real ADHD symptoms and the problems these symptoms cause in their lives and not free-floating without a specific focus as in generalized anxiety disorder.

25. When anxiety and ADHD occur together, should the anxiety or the ADHD be treated first or should they be treated at the same time?

When ADHD and anxiety occur together, it is important to first try to determine if the anxiety is a true coexisting condition or whether it is the result of ADHD symptoms. Women and girls with coexisting anxiety often cannot identify which disorder is causing them the most difficulty. Treatment of the ADHD symptoms can often make the picture clearer. For many of these girls and women, their anxiety will decrease with the reduction of their ADHD symptoms. So, if treating the ADHD with a stimulant improves the ADHD symptoms and lessens the anxiety, the anxiety was most likely the result of the untreated ADHD.

However, if upon treating the ADHD with stimulants, the anxiety stays the same or worsens, then the anxiety should be considered a separate disorder that may need to be treated in addition to the ADHD. Recently, the nonstimulant, **atomoxetine** (Strattera), has been used to treat ADHD with coexisting anxiety with resulting improvement of both conditions.

How do you treat anxiety that remains after treating the ADHD? A number of studies have looked at treatment of anxiety and ADHD in children. In one study conducted at the New York University (NYU) Child Study Center, children aged 6 to 17 years diagnosed with both ADHD and anxiety were treated with an optimal dose of stimulant medication (methylphenidate) for their ADHD. Eighty-one percent of this group had their ADHD symptoms improve. Children with improved ADHD, but who remained anxious, were then treated with fluvoxamine (Luvox), an antidepressant that is widely prescribed to treat major depression and anxiety disorders, or a placebo for an additional 8 weeks. When the anxiety symptoms were reassessed, no differences were found. In another study of children with ADHD treated with **methylphenidate** who also exhibited anxiety, it was found that behavior therapy significantly reduced the symptoms of anxiety (March et al., 2000). Although **psychosocial treatment** is not a **first-line treatment** for uncomplicated ADHD, it has proven to have significant benefits for children with ADHD and coexisting anxiety disorders

No studies have looked at the treatment of adults with ADHD and coexisting anxiety disorder. However, one study did track the levels of anxiety in 31 adults taking medication for ADHD, some of who received cognitive-behavioral therapy (CBT) (Safren et al., 2005).

Adults who received CBT reported lower anxiety scores. This finding suggests that in addition to medication to treat the ADHD, the anxiety symptoms may be addressed separately by using this intervention.

26. Can significant traumas early in life precipitate ADHD?

The symptoms of someone who has experienced an early **trauma** are extremely difficult to distinguish from those of ADHD; because of this similarity, a diagnosis based on a behavioral assessment alone is extremely challenging. In response to repeated trauma, a girl without ADHD, in an effort to protect herself, often becomes attuned to adult behaviors that may be threatening or lead to violence. Hypervigilance allows this girl to scan her environment for threats. This hypervigilance can mimic hyperactivity or inattentiveness in school because she is more focused on distractions like the teacher's face or another child's movements than her schoolwork. A door slamming closed may trigger a fight-or-flight response that a teacher may perceive as aggressive or defiant. Since both ADHD and trauma result in strikingly similar behaviors, it makes sense that some victims of early trauma are incorrectly diagnosed as having ADHD.

Abuse is, however, commonly seen in the history of girls with ADHD. In one study of a diverse population of girls aged 6 to 12 years with ADHD compared to girls without ADHD, there were significantly higher rates of previous childhood abuse for girls with ADHD (14.3%) than for the comparison sample (4.5%), with most of the abuse found in girls with combined as opposed to the inattentive subtype (Briscoe-Smith & Hinshaw, 2006). While it makes sense that when the two conditions co-occur, they would exacerbate one another, making the situation worse. There is no research that demonstrates this hypothesis at this time.

27. Are girls with ADHD more oppositional than boys with ADHD or girls without the disorder?

Just ask the mother of a daughter with ADHD and you will have the answer to this question! Oppositional defiant disorder is commonly seen in conjunction with ADHD, but much more commonly in boys. In most studies, the incidence of oppositional defiant disorder is reported to be anywhere from 40% to 60% in males and from 20% to 24% in females with ADHD. In Hinshaw's study of girls with ADHD, conducted in 2002, however, **oppositional behaviors** were reported in 71% of girls with combined subtype ADHD and 47% of the inattentive subtype compared to 7% of the girls without ADHD. Why are these percentages so high, when compared to results from other studies? While it is only a hypothesis, the answer to this question may lie in the setting for this research.

The study was carried out during a 5-week summer camp program and ratings were made while the girls were off medication. The majority, if not all, of the questionnaires assessing oppositional behaviors were completed by the girls' mothers. The phenomenon of increased responses indicating oppositional behaviors could thus conceivably be accounted for by the negative interactions occurring between mother and daughter around various issues or in situations when ADHD behaviors predominate because the ADHD is untreated. During the summer months, when a girl is not in school and/or her ADHD symptoms are not being controlled with medication, the day-to-day situations created by ADHD can quickly become toxic to any relationship, but it seems that the mother/daughter **dyad** is particularly susceptible to this scenario.

28. What is the toxic mother/daughter dyad?

In our book, *Understanding Girls with AD/HD* (2001), Drs. Nadeau, Littman, and I refer, for the first time, to the **toxic mother/daughter dyad**. There, we described the negative pattern of interactions frequently seen between mother and daughter when the daughter has ADHD. It seems that when presented with the difficulties her daughter's ADHD symptoms create, a mother becomes hypercritical of her daughter's behavior and the daughter often becomes oppositional—to her mother only. Mothers expect their daughters to have self-control and to be responsible, neat, and organized. Mothers understand, firsthand, how critical these attributes are for a woman to function and be successful on a daily basis. When they see their daughters unable to live up to expectations because of their ADHD symptoms, mothers become frightened and worry about how their daughters will succeed in the world. This fear and anxiety often translates into constant criticism and negative interactions.

Girls with ADHD also behave in ways that contribute to this toxic relationship. As discussed in the answer to Question 27 regarding oppositional behaviors, girls with ADHD often take a negative position when engaging in interactions with their mothers, fueling this vicious cycle of conflict. Girls with ADHD often have difficulty expressing themselves verbally as a result of language organization and retrieval problems. Instead of talking, they act out by slamming doors, by yelling, or with temper tantrums. For girls with ADHD, any topic or situation may become the tinder that sets off an explosive outburst.

For girls with ADHD, any topic or situation may become the tinder that sets off an explosive outburst.

This cycle of criticism and conflict, rather than the symptoms of ADHD, is often the cause of a great deal of the shame girls with ADHD experience as they grow up. Therefore, it is critical that both mothers and daughters understand the dynamics of these potentially damaging interactions. Holding important discussions only when your daughter's medication is working should diminish some of this emotional reactivity. This simple step may help your daughter to gain control of her emotions and to slow down enough to organize what she is really trying to say. In addition, allowing your daughter time to process and formulate her thoughts prior to a discussion may facilitate better communication. Behaviors exhibited when your daughter is off medication are most likely the result of her ADHD, not an innate desire to undermine your relationship. Keeping this in mind may allow you to have more patience with your daughter and to view these situations as opportunities for growth rather than conflict.

What Can a Mother Do to Break This Cycle?

If you are the mother of a daughter with ADHD and find yourself entrenched in a negative relationship with her, it is critical that you seek the help of a mental health professional who can assist you in reducing the conflict level in your relationship with your daughter. In addition to understanding how ADHD affects your daughter on a daily basis, it is also important to work on helping her improve her communication and problem-solving skills. As a mother, you play a critical role in helping your daughter understand her ADHD and learn more effective ways to deal with it on a daily basis. Your daughter will receive enough negative criticism from those who do not fully understand her ADHD. She needs you to help her cope with her

As a mother, you play a critical role in helping your daughter understand her ADHD.

ADHD challenges and recognize her many talents and strengths. Frequently, having realistic goals and setting appropriate expectations for your daughter will be the keys to improving your relationship and freeing you from the toxic mother/daughter dyad.

29. Can a person with ADHD also have a learning disability?

If you use the DSM-IV–based criteria for learning disorders, which are based on a model where a discrepancy is seen between actual achievement and prediction of achievement based on your cognitive ability or IQ, it appears that the ADHD co-occurs with learning disabilities about 20% to 30% of the time. However, it should be noted that some other studies have reported much higher rates of learning disorders (up to 70%) occurring with ADHD. These studies, however, did not follow DSM-IV criteria for a specific learning disorder and typically based the diagnosis on much looser criteria. That being said, it is important to emphasize that all students with ADHD have problems learning. Their attention and executive functioning deficits certainly affect academic achievement on a daily basis. Careless mistakes and memory deficits impair learning and recall of information resulting in poor test performance. Organizational problems impact both writing and verbal skills. And, while no specific reading disability may be diagnosed, reading comprehension can be affected if a student is not paying attention to what she is reading.

All students with ADHD have problems learning.

Treatment for ADHD, while having no impact on documented specific learning disabilities, can improve academic achievement (grades) in students with the learning deficits by reducing ADHD symptoms. Recent studies have documented that stimulants work as well in students with ADHD and learning disabilities as they do in students with ADHD only.

30. Is there a connection between ADHD and fibromyalgia?

Fibromyalgia is a poorly understood, chronic musculoskeletal condition causing widespread pain, fatigue, and muscle stiffness throughout the body. Over the years, clinicians have noticed that certain patients with ADHD, typically those with inattentive symptoms, regularly complain of fatigue and widespread musculoskeletal pain. Many of these women already have a diagnosis of fibromyalgia or chronic fatigue. In his book, *AD/HD Grown Up: A Guide to Adolescent and Adult AD/HD*, Dr. Joel Young (2007) discusses this observation and has proposed that a lifelong history of ADHD may predispose women to various chronic pain syndromes, including fibromyalgia, chronic fatigue, vulvodynia, and irritable bowel syndrome. He observes that the natural disease progression for some patients with ADHD leads to the development of chronic fatigue or fibromyalgia, whereas patients with ADHD hyperactive type may be more likely to develop restless legs syndrome (RLS) (see further discussion on RLS in Question 88). Other clinicians have reported the same findings and further go on to discuss that when the ADHD is treated with a stimulant, the pain of fibromyalgia also decreases.

Fibromyalgia research has implicated low levels of dopamine as a cause for the disorder. A study in 1998 by Krause, Krause, Magyarosy, Ernst, and Pongratz was the first to document what physicians had been seeing. They found that many cases of fibromyalgia responded well to treatment with the stimulants used to threat ADHD. It is postulated that treatment with

Certain patients with ADHD, typically those with inattentive symptoms, regularly complain of fatigue and widespread musculoskeletal pain.

stimulants by increasing dopamine and norepinephrine levels arouse patients with fatigue or allow patients with fibromyalgia and ADHD to filter out extraneous stimuli and raise the pain threshold, thus decreasing the pain. I have worked with many women who report that they become acutely aware of when their ADHD medications wear off because their fibromyalgia pain returns at the same time. This ADHD–fibromyalgia/chronic fatigue connection and its treatment have been well documented by Patricia Stephens, a certified nutrition consultant, and are addressed on both her Web site: www.addfibro.com; and in her 2010 book, *Reversing Chronic Disease: A Journey Back to Health*.

31. Why do some girls with ADHD have problems adjusting to certain noises, clothes, and foods, and what can be done about it?

In addition to other better known conditions, some girls (and women) with ADHD may also have coexisting **sensory integration dysfunction**. While not as common or well-known as anxiety, depression, or learning disabilities, the presence of sensory integration dysfunction can be just as bothersome and extremely upsetting to family life and routines. Sensory integration dysfunction can best be understood in terms of its name—that is, a disorder caused by the brain's difficulty (dysfunction) processing and integrating stimuli (touch, light, sound, and smells) as they come in from the outside world through our senses. To better understand the impact of this disorder, let's discuss each sensation in turn.

Touch

Difficulty processing touch creates considerable problems for girls with sensory integration dysfunction in many ways. Rough fabrics, tags, tight waistbands, and seams in socks are just a few of the noxious items that bother these girls and that make dressing or undressing a nightmare in many households. Likewise, hair washing and bath time may be upsetting as these girls react negatively to the water touching their skin or face. Taste, texture, and smell sensitivities make food, eating, and mealtimes a challenge as well. Girls with sensory integration issues may accept only a limited number of foods that are characteristically soft, bland, and not too hot, cold, or spicy. Eating behaviors often become a source of conflict in many homes as girls will eat only a very limited variety of foods, for example, macaroni, soup, bagels, applesauce, yogurt, cereal, and so forth. Allowing your daughter to choose her diet within reason and to provide supplements when necessary is often the only way to cope with this issue until her brain matures.

Sound

Girls with ADHD may also be very sensitive to sounds and noises, often hearing sounds that others tune out. A heating fan whirring in the background, a ticking clock, or the humming of fluorescent lighting may be quite upsetting and distracting for these girls. Parties or noisy events in large rooms with lots of people (cafeteria at school, stores, or family gatherings) may disorient them because of the buzz of conversation and high level of background noise. Sudden, loud noises may be alarming as well as disorienting.

Dealing with Sensory Integration Problems

By observing your daughter, you will be better able to distinguish what seems to bother her the most and take steps to help her avoid or process these stimuli better. For example, if she has trouble having her hair washed, letting her pour the water over her head may help. Showers may be more tolerable than baths or vice versa.

Soft clothes without tags and elastic waistbands may be all that your daughter is willing to wear. By providing her with an acceptable wardrobe made up of clothes that you know she will tolerate and wear, you may be able to salvage calm in the morning or at bedtime. Headphones may be worn (with or without music) to filter out distracting noises, and preparing your daughter ahead of time for large crowds may help somewhat. In addition, if problems become unmanageable or your daughter seems to need more help, I suggest you seek out the services of a certified occupational therapist (OT) trained to deal with this disorder. An OT will be able to set up a program to help you work on problem areas and desensitize your daughter to these noxious stimuli.

32. Are girls and women with ADHD at risk for developing eating disorders?

The recent discovery of the association between **eating disorders** and ADHD can have significant implications for women and girls with ADHD. Unfortunately, this critical link has been overlooked for too long and has come into the spotlight only recently for several reasons. Most of the early studies of ADHD were conducted using male-only populations or in preadolescents—two groups where the incidence of eating pathology is low. Unfortunately, it was not until we started following females with ADHD into adolescence that this link became apparent. A higher incidence of eating disorders in adult women with ADHD was also recently noted, but only when data was examined retrospectively.

The ADHD/disordered eating connection is not difficult to understand. Eating disorders and ADHD share several key characteristics, including impulsivity

Women and girls with ADHD develop eating disorders for many reasons.

(lack of **self-regulation**), depression, and low self-esteem. However, women and girls with ADHD develop eating disorders for many reasons. Symptoms of ADHD can contribute to the development of **binge eating** and other disordered eating patterns as a woman loses her ability to control what she eats and how she responds to events in her environment. Many women with ADHD eat for stimulation or to feel better. Others get distracted, forget to eat, and then have no control once they impulsively start eating. These eating patterns often result in chronic overeating and obesity as women have no idea of how many calories they are consuming each day. When two samples of adults with and without ADHD were retrospectively examined, significantly greater rates of **bulimia nervosa** were identified in women with ADHD versus those without ADHD (12% vs. 3% for one sample and 11% vs. 1%, for the other sample). Although preliminary and requiring further confirmation, these findings suggest that bulimia nervosa may be associated with ADHD in some women.

Two studies of adolescent girls previously diagnosed with ADHD also found a significant incidence of eating disorders (Biederman et al., 2007; Mikami et al., 2008). In the first study of adolescent girls with and without ADHD found that those with ADHD were 3.6 times more likely to develop an eating disorder, defined as either **anorexia** or bulimia nervosa. During the study's 5-year follow-up, 16% of the girls with ADHD (20 girls) and 5% of the control subjects (5 girls) developed an eating disorder. Compared with the control subjects, the girls with ADHD were 5.6 times more likely to develop bulimia and 2.7 times more likely to develop **anorexia nervosa**. These girls with ADHD also had significantly higher rates of depression, anxiety disorders, and disruptive behavior. Occasionally, I have seen girls with ADHD and anxiety, who stop eating as a means of controlling a world that they see as being out of their control. Few, however, develop full-blown anorexia nervosa. Usually, these girls continue to maintain an appropriate body image and they do not develop a drive for thinness; they simply want to gain an element of control.

In the second study, 93 adolescent girls with ADHD-combined subtype, 49 with ADHD-inattentive subtype, and 88 girls without ADHD were assessed for eating disorders (Mikami et al., 2008). In this study, baseline impulsivity symptoms best predicted adolescent eating abnormalities, as did the diagnosis of ADHD-combined subtype. In addition, peer rejection and parent–child relationship patterns were seen as predictive of eating disorders in the girls with ADHD.

Treatment for many of the eating patterns described earlier may be accomplished by treating the ADHD symptoms that underlie them. In an article published in the May 2005 issue of the *Journal of Women's Health*, Dr. Carolyn Dukarm, an eating disorder specialist, described six patients with bulimia and ADHD who were treated with dextroamphetamine. All six patients reported no further episodes of binge eating and purging following treatment. In five of the six patients, ADHD had not been previously diagnosed, perhaps due to the fact that all six had the inattentive subtype of the disorder. These cases, along with the recent clinical study findings seem to confirm the association between bulimia nervosa/binge eating and ADHD in girls and women, and have important clinical and treatment implications. In 2006, Dr. Dukarm presented a

Some girls with ADHD and anxiety stop eating as a means of controlling a world that they see as being out of their control.

more detailed look at the potential role of ADHD and its treatment in the management of women with bulimia. In *Pieces of a Puzzle: The Link Between ADHD and Eating Disorders*, Dr. Dukarm offers an extremely detailed diagnosis and treatment program for patients with the dual diagnosis and for the clinicians who treat them.

PART THREE

Treatment of ADHD in Girls and Women

How can I help my daughter deal with her ADHD?

What is the ideal dose or medication
to treat ADHD?

Should ADHD be treated throughout the
day and into the evening? What about weekends
and holidays?

More . . .

33. What constitutes the best treatment for ADHD in women and girls?

Treatment with various medications that work by regulating the neurotransmitter systems in the brain thereby reducing ADHD symptoms continues to be the first-line and best treatment for ADHD for both males and females. In fact, many women and girls with relatively mild and uncomplicated cases of ADHD may respond well to drug therapy alone. However, even if a woman is fortunate enough to be correctly diagnosed with ADHD, treatment regimens are usually made up of recommendations established by those experienced in treating elementary school-aged boys.

If you are considering taking medication for your ADHD, be sure to work with an experienced and knowledgeable physician who can guide you in the correct administration and dosing of the various stimulant or **nonstimulant medications** used to control ADHD symptoms. Treatment with medication should always follow a careful evaluation including medical, psychiatric, social, and cognitive assessments. Although improvement in the symptoms of ADHD provided by these medications can be impressive, these changes will not necessarily translate into satisfactory functional improvements in your daily life in areas such as self-esteem, time management, organization, and interpersonal relationships. Thus, you might need a combination of several treatment approaches and support services or a **multimodal treatment** approach, designed specifically to meet your diverse needs.

Girls with ADHD stand to benefit from medication management of their ADHD symptoms as much as boys, but certain differences need to be considered. In addition to treating ADHD symptoms, the low

Girls with ADHD stand to benefit from medication management of their ADHD symptoms as much as boys, but certain differences need to be considered.

self-esteem, shame, demoralization, and negative thoughts that accompany ADHD in these girls may need to be addressed in individual psychotherapy or cognitive-behavioral therapy. Girls are more likely to internalize symptoms and become anxious, depressed, and socially withdrawn. These feelings, experienced as early as age 8 or 9, tend to intensify as a girl moves through middle school and into high school, and require a coordinated treatment approach in order to improve overall functioning and prevent negative behaviors. In some cases, untreated ADHD may lead to substance abuse disorders and sexual acting out behaviors as these girls enter adolescence, and these behaviors are not without repercussions. Even many years after such adolescent acting out, women with ADHD often report feelings of shame and self-blame for the behaviors they exhibited during these years.

For women with ADHD, issues relating to depression, anxiety, low self-esteem, social rejection and/or isolation, and struggles as a wife and mother to live up to society's expectations, not to mention the impossible demands of single motherhood, may need to be addressed in individual psychotherapy or cognitive behavioral therapy (CBT). In addition, the struggles with daily life management and organization may call for women with ADHD to work with an ADHD coach and/or professional organizer. Overall for best results, ADHD in women should be viewed as a complicated disorder requiring a complex treatment program.

34. How can I help my daughter deal with her ADHD?

Girls with ADHD can be challenging; the key to success, however, is often the understanding and support they receive at home. The issues faced by girls with

In some cases, untreated ADHD may lead to substance abuse disorders and sexual acting out behaviors as these girls enter adolescence.

ADHD are clearly very different from those of typical elementary school-aged boys with the disorder. To help your daughter with ADHD, it is critical that you understand these issues, often based on her ADHD subtype diagnosis.

In addition to her ADHD, a girl with inattentive subtype may exhibit problems both socially and emotionally. The rapid give and take of group interactions may prove difficult for her. She may act shy or feel socially out of it except with one best friend. In addition, a **hypersensitivity** to criticism from parents and others may develop. At school, she may demonstrate a desire to conform to teacher expectations and not draw attention to herself. Yet, all too often, her distractibility or forgetfulness results in teacher disapproval and/or embarrassment and humiliation in front of her peers.

Her hyperactive/impulsive subtype counterpart has different problems altogether. Life for this girl can be an emotional roller coaster. In addition to being hyperactive, she can be stubborn, angry, defiant, and rebellious. She can be hyperreactive as well as hyperemotional. Her low frustration tolerance and disorganization can lead to a great deal of stress for her and others.

Adolescence is a difficult time for all girls, but add ADHD to the mix, and everyday problems and stresses become amplified. A girl with ADHD who may have been coping because she received a great deal of support during the early years may become overwhelmed. For the hyperactive, hyperemotional girl, life provides more opportunities for high stimulation with the accompanying higher risks as she enters adolescence. So, how can you help these girls?

Ways to Help Your Daughter with ADHD

Provide Her with a Safe Space to Time-Out, Relax, and Regain Control

Whether she is shy and withdrawn or hyper and impulsive, a girl with ADHD often feels emotionally overwhelmed. To regain control, your daughter needs to learn to recognize what pushes her buttons and to avoid these situations or people instead of succumbing to her emotions. In addition, she needs to become familiar with the signs of stress in her body and develop a set of stress management techniques. Even when she is very young, you can impress upon her the value of taking an emotional **time-out**, not as a punishment, but as a way to regroup after an emotional upset. By helping her set up a safe, quiet place in her room or elsewhere in your home that she can use as a retreat when things get difficult, you will encourage her to take steps to gain greater self-control over her emotions and her ADHD.

Minimize Corrections and Criticism

Often in an attempt to help their daughter overcome her disability, parents fall into the trap of continually pointing out her failures. Girls with ADHD are usually in a great deal of pain and burdened by shame as it is. Correction and criticism only add to that burden. In addition, girls can be oppositional and negative when interacting with their mothers as part of the toxic mother/daughter dyad (see Question 28 on page 47 for a more in-depth discussion of this relationship). That being said, I want to make it clear that I'm not advocating a complete hands-off approach. What I am advocating is an attempt to be more empathetic and sensitive to your daughter's needs. A kind word at the end of a difficult day at school or an understanding pat on the shoulder or hug when she knows she has made a mess of something can often be more effective than pointing out what went wrong. Often by asking questions rather than criticizing, you will find that you open up rather than shut down the lines of communication and provide opportunities for change. Your daughter is most likely very aware of the situation. A simple, "How old are you acting right now?" rather than a "Stop spinning in that chair!" may be all that is needed to help your daughter change her behavior. An "It must be difficult when _____ happens," rather than a "You've messed up again!" is so much more effective and preserves, rather than erodes, her self-esteem.

Help Your Daughter Find Her "Islands of Competence"

Girls with ADHD often feel that they are not good at anything. They tend to give up easily and may have difficulty developing their skills or focusing on their talents. By helping your daughter discover her strengths and establishing an "island" or activity where she feels competent, you can help build her self-concept as well as improve her self-esteem. By recognizing and praising her for her efforts, not just her accomplishments, you will encourage her to attempt new activities and boost her self-confidence. Over the years, I have often seen girls with ADHD, who have previously experienced a great deal of heartbreak because of their poor social skills, blossom as they discover their untapped ability to work with younger children, seniors, or animals.

35. What medications are used to treat ADHD in women and girls?

Research and clinical experience have shown that stimulant medications are the most effective first-line treatment for ADHD in both males and females.

Currently, there are many medication formulations, including stimulants (methylphenidate and **amphetamine** preparations) and nonstimulants for the treatment of ADHD. Although a few skeptics continue to voice concerns over the prescription of medication for children and adults with ADHD, studies suggest that stimulant medication is the most effective treatment option for ADHD and that, in some studies in children, medication alone has a positive treatment effect equal to medication in combination with behavior therapy.

Most patients respond equally well to either methylphenidate or amphetamine preparations. While early studies on the effectiveness of medications to treat ADHD were conducted solely on young boys, more recent studies have included women and girls with the disorder, who have responded as well as males to both stimulants and nonstimulants. Given the high variability in **effective dose** for each individual, however, when undertaking treatment of ADHD with stimulants or nonstimulants, a person should be started at the lowest dose possible and the dosage increased every 5 to 7 days until effective symptom reduction and normalization of functioning is achieved.

Methylphenidate Preparations

Methylphenidate products for the treatment of ADHD include the well-known brand, **Ritalin**, an **immediate-release preparation** that takes effect in a relatively short period of time and lasts about 4 hours. Ritalin is also available as long-acting formulation Ritalin LA. Other long-acting medications containing methylphenidate include Concerta, Focalin XR, Daytrana, Metadate CD, and Methylin.

Amphetamine Preparations

Both **Dexedrine**, **Adderall**, and **Vyvanse** are trade names for products whose active component is a formulation of amphetamine or amphetamine salts. Dexedrine, which has been available for many years, is equally as effective as methylphenidate for a number of problems associated with ADHD, but is not prescribed as frequently. Adderall is the trade name for a generic compound of mixed amphetamine salts (three forms of d-amphetamine and one of l-amphetamine). Adderall, which has been studied in children, has been shown to be effective in reducing disruptive behaviors in a classroom setting, improving parent and teacher behavior ratings, and improving academic performance. It is recommended that the maximum daily dose not exceed 40 mg. The duration of effects of Adderall is generally dose-dependent, with higher doses resulting in longer duration of action (e.g., 5 mg is usually effective for 3.52 hours, and 20 mg usually produces effects for 6.4 hours). Adderall is also available as a once-daily formulation (called Adderall XR), which has a much longer duration of action (10 to 12 hours). Vyvanse is a newer long-acting drug formulation. Vyvanse is one of the longest-acting stimulant formulations on the market and has a low likelihood of abuse since the drug is not active until it is broken down in the body.

Nonstimulants

In addition to the first-line stimulants, **nonstimulants** have also been prescribed to treat ADHD, usually as an off-label use or **second-line therapy**. These nonstimulants include imipramine (Tofranil), desipramine (Norpramin), bupropion (Wellbutrin), venlafaxine (Effexor), **clonidine** (Catapres), **guanfacine** (Tenex), and modafinil

(Provigil). In the past, however, these medications have never been quite as effective as stimulants and were used off-label, not having received Food and Drug Administration (FDA) approval for the treatment of ADHD.

Intuniv

Recently, a once-daily, extended-release formulation of Intuniv (guanfacine) has been approved for the treatment of ADHD in children and adolescents. In clinical trials, Intuniv demonstrated significant reduction in both ADHD and oppositional symptoms. Intuniv is not a controlled substance and has no known mechanism for abuse or dependence. The most common side effect of this drug is sedation, which is usually transient and mild to moderate in severity. Fainting occurred in approximately 1% of pediatric patients in the clinical trials. Small to modest changes in blood pressure, pulse rate, and electrocardiogram parameters were also observed.

Strattera

In 2004, atomoxetine (Strattera), another nonstimulant, was approved for the treatment of ADHD. Full therapeutic effects of atomoxetine may take at least a week to be felt, but once adequate blood levels are obtained, effectiveness can last for 24 hours. Therefore. atomoxetine should be taken for 6 to 8 weeks before you decide whether it is working or not. Some people who do not respond to stimulants respond to atomoxetine. Atomoxetine has a low potential for abuse and is not a controlled substance.

Table 2 lists medications (stimulants and nonstimulants) used to treat ADHD, their duration of action, and a brief description of each.

Table 2   Stimulants

Methylphenidate Class		
Immediate-Release *Duration 3–4 hours*	**Description**	**Dosages Available**
Ritalin	Methylphenidate	5 mg, 10 mg, and 20 mg
Focalin	Refined form of Ritalin, isolating the *d*-isomer	2.5 mg, 5 mg, and 10 mg
Methylin	Methylphenidate	5 mg, 10 mg, and 20 mg
Methylin chewables	Chewable methylphenidate	2.5 mg, 5 mg, and 10 mg
Methylin suspension	Liquid methylphenidate	5 mg/5 ml and 10 mg/5 ml
Long-Acting *Duration 8–12 hours*	**Description IM/ER Ratio***	**Dosages Available**
Ritalin SR	Methylphenidate 50/50	20 mg
Ritalin LA	Methylphenidate 50/50, mimics twice a day dosing	10 mg, 20 mg, 30 mg, and 40 mg
Metadate CD	Methylphenidate 30/70	10 mg, 20 mg, 30 mg, 40 mg, 50 mg, and 60 mg
Concerta	Methylphenidate 22/78, mimics 3x a day dosing	18 mg, 27 mg, 36 mg, and 54 mg
Focalin XR	Dextromethylphenidate 50/50	5 mg, 10 mg, 15 mg, and 20 mg
Methylin ER	Methylphenidate 50/50	10 mg and 20 mg
Daytrana	Methylphenidate Transdermal patch delivering 1.1/1.6/2.2/3.3 mg/hr over 9 hours	10 mg, 15 mg, 20 mg, and 30 mg
Amphetamine Class		
Immediate-Release *Duration 4–5 hours*	**Description**	**Dosages Available**
Dexedrine	Dextroamphetamine	5 mg and 10 mg
Adderall	Mixed amphetamine salts	5 mg, 7.5 mg, 10 mg, 12.5 mg, 15 mg, 20 mg, and 30 mg

*Immediate Release/Extended Release Ratio

Long-Acting *Duration 8–14 hours*	Description	Dosages Available
Adderall XR	Mixed amphetamine salts, mimics twice a day dose	5 mg, 10 mg, 15 mg, 20 mg, 25 mg, and 30 mg
Dexedrine Spansule	Dextroamphetamine	5 mg, 10 mg, and 15 mg
Vyvanse	Lisdexamfetamine (a prodrug activated in the body)	20 mg, 30 mg, 40 mg, 50 mg, 60 mg, and 70 mg
Nonstimulants		
Long-Acting *Duration 24 hours*	Description	Dosage Available
Strattera	Atomoxetine	10 mg, 18 mg, 25 mg, 40 mg, 60 mg, 80 mg, and 100 mg
Intuniv	Guanfacine	1 mg, 2 mg, 3 mg, and 4 mg

Treatment of ADHD in Girls and Women

Medications Approved for Adults with ADHD

Although widely used in adults, only a few of these medications have been formally approved by the FDA for use in adults with ADHD. Since 2004, the following medications have been approved for the treatment of ADHD in adults: the nonstimulant Strattera (atomoxetine), Adderall XR (mixed amphetamine salts), Vyvanse (lisdexamfetamine), **Focalin** XR (dextromethylphenidate), and **Concerta** (methylphenidate). In addition to these medications, a few clinical trials have shown that **Provigil** (modafinil), a waking agent used for the treatment of excessive daytime sleepiness; **Wellbutrin** (buproprion); **Tofranil** (imipramine); and **Norpramin** (desipramine) can be somewhat effective, although none of these medications is specifically approved for the treatment of ADHD.

Effectiveness of Medications to Treat ADHD

The ability of stimulants to treat ADHD is excellent; most are at least 70% effective when prescribed at appropriate dosages in adults. Studies that have looked at the effects of gender on the response to stimulants in women have not shown any difference in efficacy or safety. At higher doses, as many as 80% of adults respond to stimulants with a decrease in symptoms seen as early as the first week of treatment. Nonstimulants, (Strattera and Intuniv) are also quite effective but at slightly lower rates.

36. What is the ideal dose of medication to treat ADHD?

In general, an ideal or optimum dose of medication is the one at which a person's ADHD symptoms are optimally controlled and her overall functioning is normalized (rated as being within the same range of people without ADHD) with any side effects being kept at a tolerable level. So, how does one achieve this balance? The primary means to accomplish this end is to individualize treatment. Your treating physician will most likely start you on the lowest recommended dose of a particular medication. The dose will then be increased in small increments every week or so while your physician continuously monitors the medication's effects on targeted symptoms, and at the same time inquiring about side effects. Higher doses are more likely to provide optimum results. Side effects, however, may occur at any dose level and are usually mild to moderate (see Question 46 for a discussion on side effects) and diminish over time. The ultimate dose of medication, in general, and stimulants, in particular, is not based on weight or age, but rather on an individual's needs and response during a well-controlled trial. It is important for you to work closely with your physician to get the best results from your treatment.

37. Are some medications more effective in treating ADHD in women than in men?

Several studies have demonstrated that medications are highly effective in the treatment of ADHD symptoms in adult patients, whether male or female. In fact, many adult patients with uncomplicated cases of ADHD respond well to drug therapy alone. Medication issues for women with ADHD, however, are often more complicated than those for men for a number of reasons. First, as discussed previously, women with ADHD are more likely to suffer from coexisting anxiety and/or depression, as well as a range of other conditions. Alcohol and drug use disorders, often beginning at an early age, are frequently encountered in women with ADHD, so if you have a history of such disorders, it is very important to discuss them with your doctor prior to treatment for ADHD. However, while substance abuse may complicate the picture, it should in no way deter your clinician from prescribing appropriate treatment for ADHD. In fact, it may be the treatment of your ADHD that allows you to stay in recovery from various addictions.

To further complicate the picture, women with ADHD may suffer from various medical conditions, including **hypothyroidism, fibromyalgia, chronic fatigue syndrome**, and eating disorders. Therefore, an effective medication approach for a woman with ADHD needs to take into consideration all aspects of her life including the treatment of coexisting conditions, addictions, and other medical issues, as well as her ADHD.

Second, medicating women with ADHD may be further complicated by **hormone** fluctuations across the **menstrual cycle** and across the life span (e.g., **puberty, perimenopause**, and **menopause**) with an increase in ADHD symptoms whenever estrogen levels fall. In some cases, because of worsening symptoms, a woman with ADHD might also need to consider **hormone replacement therapy**. (See Questions 72 and 73 for a more in-depth discussion on the relationship between hormones and ADHD symptoms in women.) Little is known about the interactions between hormones and stimulant medications. While ADHD symptoms respond to stimulant medication in both females and in males, hormone levels during certain phases of the cycle may, however, decrease their effectiveness. Cyclical variations of hormones (both **estrogen** and **progesterone**) during the menstrual cycle often need to be considered in determining the proper dose of medication for women.

Medication is the only treatment for ADHD that works primarily by altering the underlying abnormalities in the brain's neurotransmitters.

38. How do I know if my medications are working?

Medication is the only treatment for ADHD that works primarily by altering the underlying abnormalities in the brain's neurotransmitters. It is easy to determine if your medication is working if you know what to look for. But keep in mind that for your medication to work, you need to take it as prescribed by your physician. Be sure to take your medication every day at the time and dose prescribed. If you have difficulty remembering to take a dose, work with your physician or ADHD coach to develop an effective reminder system such as setting a watch alarm or establishing a link between taking a pill and an external cue. If remembering multiple doses throughout the day is problematic, ask your physician if one of the newer once-daily formulations or a patch would be a better option for you.

Once you are correctly and consistently taking your medication, it is time to assess how well it is working. As part of the evaluation you underwent to make the diagnosis of ADHD, your physician most likely asked you and/or others to complete various rating scales that looked at symptoms and everyday functioning. In addition, you may have set target symptoms to guide you and help determine the effectiveness of your treatment program. Both of these (rating scales and target symptoms) can help you determine if your medication is at the ideal dose (see Question 36 for a further discussion on the ideal dose) to provide an optimum response.

The main goals of treating ADHD are to reduce symptoms and normalize functioning. Instead of subjectively rating improvement, you and your physician can monitor your progress and determine when these goals are achieved by observing when your symptoms, as documented on rating scales, fall to within the range of scores seen in individuals without ADHD. Ratings can be made weekly, and guide the increases in dose to an optimum response. If target symptoms do not respond to increasing doses of a particular medication, you will know that medication is not working and that another medication may be necessary. A word of caution is in order here, however. Be sure that you have tried a medication for an adequate length of time and at an appropriate dosage level before you consider it a failure. I often hear from parents of girls or women with ADHD that they have tried various medications and they did not work only to find upon further questioning that they may have taken a particular medication for 1 or 2 days and stopped because they got a stomachache or that they only tried the lowest strength of a medication and that the dose was never adjusted upward. Remember, finding the right medication for you will take some time and patience.

39. When a girl or woman has ADHD and multiple coexisting conditions, what are some general guidelines for treatment? Which disorder should be treated first?

The American Academy of Child and Adolescent Psychiatry addressed this issue in a 2002 article, "Practice Parameter for the Use of Stimulant Medications in the Treatment of Children, Adolescents, and Adults." In a discussion on the treatment of ADHD with coexisting mood disorders, the article states that if ADHD is accompanied by severe symptoms of a **major depressive disorder** with **psychosis**, thoughts of suicide, or **vegetative symptoms** (not eating or decreased or excessive sleeping), treatment should be prioritized, and the depressive disorder should be treated first. If symptoms of depression are less severe (mild to moderate), there may be an advantage to treating the ADHD first. Reduction of ADHD symptoms may have a significant effect on the chronic low levels of depression or demoralization that result when ADHD goes untreated.

In fact, in most cases no other treatment will be necessary. However, if the ADHD symptoms respond and the depression remains, other treatments should be instituted. These include cognitive behavioral therapy, psychotherapy, or antidepressant medication. In addition, if a woman or girl has been treated for depression prior to her ADHD diagnosis, her depressive symptoms should be reassessed after the ADHD symptoms are under control.

When treating ADHD and anxiety, physicians should consider treating the ADHD with stimulants, first. If the stimulant improves the ADHD symptoms, but the anxiety remains, psychosocial intervention for the anxiety can then be undertaken. If the anxiety does not improve or worsens, the physician may consider adding an antianxiety medication to the treatment program at that point.

For many years, it was thought that stimulants should not be given to children with ADHD and **tics**, for fear of increasing the tics. Studies, however, have now shown that stimulants can be highly effective in the treatment of ADHD in this group, and that for the majority of these patients, tics do not increase. After explaining the risks to the patient or her family, the physician may try stimulants in these cases. If tics remain the same and ADHD symptoms respond to stimulants, the patient can then remain on the stimulants. A physician may choose at that time to treat the tics if they are problematic for the patient on a daily basis. Clonidine or guanfacine are commonly recommended for treatment of tics in these cases. However, if tics increase significantly while the patient is on stimulants, the physician should consider an alternative therapy or treating the tics first and, once they are stabilized, then adding back the stimulant (usually at a lower dose).

40. If I suspect I have ADHD, how do I find a doctor or mental health professional to diagnose and treat me? What questions should I ask to determine if that professional is knowledgeable, experienced, and enthusiastic about treating ADHD in women or girls?

Finding a mental health professional or physician with experience in diagnosing and treating women and girls with ADHD may not be an easy task in many communities. However, I have several tips and strategies I would like to share with you that may help you in this process. First, be a wise consumer. This involves interviewing professionals within your community prior to seeking their opinion regarding diagnosis or requesting treatment. Prepare a list of questions ahead of time and do not be afraid to ask them. Inquire as to the amount of training and experience in diagnosing ADHD the professional has had, and the percentage or number of women or girls diagnosed and treated in his/her practice. Ask for his/her opinions regarding ADHD in women and girls and for a list of books he/she has read about the disorder and the conferences he typically attends.

Ask others within your community for the names of professionals who have a positive reputation for treating ADHD.

Second, ask others within your community for the names of professionals who have a positive reputation for treating ADHD. Attend CHADD (Children and Adults with Attention Deficit/Hyperactivity Disorder) meetings or other community forums (some may even be local online groups) and seek out a list of professionals with knowledge of and an enthusiasm for treating ADHD in females. If you do not have a local CHADD chapter or other mental health facility, try contacting a local university's disabilities services office or the special education department of your local public schools. They should be able to tell you who they use as a referral resource for their students with suspected or confirmed ADHD. In general, in most communities, child psychiatrists may be more likely to treat ADHD than adult psychiatrists. Likewise, general practitioners and pediatricians are more likely to treat ADHD than internists. If you live near a university hospital you might also contact its departments of psychiatry or psychology for referrals. Many of these programs have mental health professionals on staff that also have private practices or run ADHD clinics. Local, state, or county mental health departments may also be able to help, but I find they are often understaffed with a long waiting time for appointments.

Last, do not expect to find one individual who can meet all of these criteria. There are few professionals in this country who can answer the majority of these questions positively. However, if you find someone who is willing to answer your questions and work with you, consider it a positive sign that you are on the right track.

Moving to a New Area

If you have already been diagnosed and undergoing treatment for some time and are planning to move, ask your current mental health professional for a list of names of professionals in your new locality and for a referral letter that you can take with you that outlines your case along with current medications including dose and the date of your last prescription. In addition, make sure that you get a copy of all of your records including medications prescribed over the years with documentation of any side effects or reasons why a particular treatment did not work. That way you will not be starting back at square one with your new physician or mental health professional.

Anna speaks:

I am a 50-year old woman diagnosed with ADD 7 years ago. I had to leave the area of the country where the MD and therapist who diagnosed me were located. I have had a very hard time finding anyone to replace my MD. Can you give me advice on how to find a knowledgeable MD? I have not had any luck using customer service at my HMO or the local mental health organization. I just need help to find the right MD. I am very frustrated as attempts to find an MD to write my prescriptions has ended several times in my being accused of drug seeking. I have never had a substance abuse problem and this prejudiced attitude is depressing and has only made my life more difficult. When it happens, I give up and muddle through with no medicine or treatment, which significantly affects my work.

41. Is it safe to take medications for the treatment of ADHD when pregnant?

To date, there have been no controlled studies in women looking at the effects of stimulants during pregnancy. There have been a few animal studies reporting **cardiac defects** at high doses of amphetamines and some individual case reports from women who took either amphetamines or methylphenidate during their pregnancies without harm to the fetus. Additional case reports indicate that women exposed to methylphenidate during pregnancy were noted to have higher than expected rates of **premature births,** growth retardation, and neonatal withdrawal in their infants. However, at this time, looking at all the available evidence, the prevailing recommendation is that stimulants should be used during pregnancy only when the potential benefits to the mother outweigh any risk to the fetus. Nonstimulants such as imipramine and clonidine have been approved for use during pregnancy so they may be an option for some women. However, a woman considering pregnancy should always discuss continuing her medication treatment for her ADHD with her prescribing physician.

42. What are some nonmedical treatment options during pregnancy?

Many women report that their ADHD symptoms seem to abate or greatly improve during pregnancy. For others, I recommend that they try **nonpharmacologic** interventions. Although these nonpharmacologic interventions are poorly studied, ADHD coaching, relaxing meditation or yoga, and cognitive behavioral therapy (CBT) may be helpful during this time. In addition, a woman should try to simplify her life and ask for help from others during her pregnancy and immediately after the birth of her child. Getting plenty of exercise, adequate rest, and enough sleep is critical as all are necessary for optimal brain functioning.

43. What are the key considerations when debating whether or not to go on medication for my ADHD?

For well over 50 years, stimulant medications have been the cornerstone of therapy to improve ADHD symptoms. Many thousands of studies have been conducted demonstrating both the safety and efficacy of stimulants.

Yet, when it comes to making a personal decision for yourself or your daughter to take one of the medications prescribed for ADHD, numerous questions invariably arise. How bad do my symptoms need to be? Will medications change my personality? Should medications be used first or as a last resort? What changes can I expect if I take medication? Once I start, will I need to take medication for the rest of my life? To answer these questions, you will need to investigate various facets of your ADHD and consider several points related to the treatment of this disorder.

Assessing how ADHD is affecting the various aspects of your life should be one of your top priorities, with special attention directed to the cost of going unmedicated. As pointed out previously, girls and women with ADHD often suffer considerable shame, depression, anxiety, and loss of self-esteem as a result of going unmedicated. Decisions to treat ADHD should be based on the degree of impairment rather than just the number or presence of certain symptoms. Research has shown that girls and women with ADHD may have fewer symptoms than males with ADHD, but that these symptoms result in the same or greater impairment.

The risks and benefits of medication should be thoroughly investigated and discussed with your treating physician before a decision to treat your ADHD is made.

The risks and benefits of medication should be thoroughly investigated and discussed with your treating physician before a decision to treat your ADHD is made. Side effects of specific medications should also be discussed and the existence of medical conditions such as heart disease or pregnancy should be ruled out before stimulants are prescribed. In addition, consideration should be given as to how the use of certain medications will affect any coexisting condition you might have. Protocols have been designed to specifically deal with these situations, but you need to be aware of and discuss these with your physician. (See Question 39 for a more in-depth discussion of treating ADHD and coexisting conditions.)

Your expectations for medication should also enter into the treatment decision. Stimulant medications have been shown to effectively reduce the core symptoms of ADHD, but they will not teach you skills or work on many of the common problems you have experienced because of your ADHD. Unfortunately, many parents of children with ADHD, as well as adults with the disorder, think that taking medications will solve all of their problems. In most cases, medications to treat ADHD should not be used alone. The availability and effectiveness of additional therapies (such as coaching, CBT, working with a professional organizer, or taking supplements) should therefore, also be considered before making a final decision.

In the end, after careful consideration of all of these aspects of the question of whether to take medications for your ADHD, one fact will remain—most individuals with ADHD need a comprehensive treatment program to effectively deal with all aspects of their ADHD, but you need to choose what is best for you.

44. Is it ever too late or can a woman be too old to start medication?

When considering whether or not to take medication, the first and most important questions to ask are not, "Is it too late?" or "Am I too old?" but instead "To what degree is ADHD affecting my life?" or "Can things be better for me?" If you need to make changes, it is never too late to consider medication therapy for your ADHD. Once you have reached the decision (in consultation with your physician) that medication therapy will be helpful in reducing your ADHD symptoms, there are some additional cautions that you should keep in mind when taking stimulants in mid- to late adulthood. These include medical, as well as psychiatric and other conditions. When starting stimulant medication therapy for patients at any age, the physician should always conduct a careful evaluation including medical, psychiatric, social, and cognitive assessments.

Aging carries with it certain inherent conditions that make the use of stimulants improper or of limited effectiveness. These include high blood pressure, glaucoma, coronary artery disease, heart failure, recent heart attack or stroke, or cardiac arrhythmias. Gastrointestinal conditions such as narrowing or **diverticula** (pouches) may increase the risk of problems with treatments of certain medications like Concerta (methylphenidate) that traverse the entire gastrointestinal tract. Older adults also have a tendency to become depressed. Assessment of mood and appropriate treatment for mood disorders should be undertaken in conjunction with an ADHD evaluation. Stimulants for the treatment of ADHD may complement or increase the efficacy of these antidepressants.

After considering these various factors, your physician will carefully tailor the choice of medication to your unique situation. Last, be sure that the goals of your therapy are clearly stated and that the risks and benefits have been completely explained to you by your physician. For best results, when setting up goals for therapy, be sure you consider your present life situation. If you are in menopause, you may need to determine the extent that the cognitive, memory, and sleep deficits commonly associated with the low levels of estrogen seen in menopause are affecting your functioning, as these are unlikely to improve with stimulants. In addition, if you are retired, you should assess how problematic the decreased structure in your life has become. Many women tell me that their ability to cope and get things done diminished greatly when they retired and no longer had the structure of work in their lives. Medication, while improving symptoms, will not provide the structure you need. Enlisting the help of a therapist or coach may be more effective in this situation.

Joanne speaks:

I am a woman who has never been formally diagnosed, but I truly believe I have ADHD. My son was diagnosed at 8 years of age. I am no stranger to the symptoms of ADHD, as I am a teacher as well. I am now 55. At this stage of the game, would there be any benefits from using medication, and if so, what problems or considerations would there be for someone my age? I don't take any medications for other reasons, but many women my age do.

45. Should ADHD be treated throughout the day and into the evening? What about weekends and holidays?

When answering this question, it is important to keep in mind that ADHD is a chronic, lifelong disorder with symptoms that can affect a person's functioning 24 hours a day, 7 days a week, 365 days a year. ADHD does not take a vacation! Remember, ADHD symptoms can affect your parenting, relationships, and even your marriage. Controlling symptoms with medication in the evenings and on weekends is often the key to improvement in these areas as well. So, when discussing treatment options with your healthcare provider and deciding whether to treat your symptoms throughout the day and on weekends, it is important to assess whether symptoms are affecting your functioning at these times. I often hear from women who report that they start to get increasingly absent-minded or non-productive in the afternoon or evening when they are coming off their medication. Medications used to treat ADHD can last varying lengths of time. Even the newer, long-acting preparations only last for approximately 12 hours—and how many women have 12 hour days?

Medications used to treat ADHD can last varying lengths of time.

What About Sleep?

Many women already have difficulty falling asleep, and **insomnia** can be a side effect of stimulants. To answer this question, it is important to determine if sleep issues were part of the ADHD and present prior to its treatment. As discussed in Question 88, many women with ADHD have problems going to sleep. These issues are the result of untreated ADHD, and if your medication has worn off by bedtime, it is likely that you are not sleeping for that reason, rather than as a side effect of treatment. Making sure that your ADHD symptoms are under control may be the best way to ensure that you will be able to fall asleep at night. Many women with ADHD also report that they are more efficient at completing tasks in the evening when on medication, and that they are then able to get to bed at a more reasonable hour, rather than needing to stay up late to get everything done as they had done previously. Getting to bed and experiencing a better night's sleep when on medication during the evening hours may be critical to improving performance the following day, thus, setting you up for a better, less sleepy, and stressful morning routine.

46. What are the most common side effects of medications used to treat ADHD?

The following is a list of the most common **side effects** of the stimulant medications:

- Headache
- Decreased appetite
- Stomachache
- Nervousness
- Trouble sleeping (insomnia)
- Dizziness
- Dry mouth

These side effects do not occur in everyone taking a stimulant medication, and even if they do occur, they tend to be short-lived and decrease over the first several months of therapy. In various studies, these side effects were found to occur in 4% to 10% of individuals treated. Serious side effects were reported to be very rare, and studies have found no differences in these side effects among the different stimulants.

In addition to the mild to moderate side effects listed earlier, more serious side effects include slowing of **growth** with continuous use over many years. However, studies have shown that height differences over time between those treated with stimulants and the control groups were minimal if at all. Recent 10-year follow-up studies of children, who have taken stimulant medications for varying lengths of time during that period, have not found any ultimate height differences. **Seizures** at high doses of stimulants or the antidepressant, Wellbutrin, used off-label to treat ADHD have been noted in patients with a history of seizures; however, these **breakthrough seizures** are rare in patients

More serious side effects include slowing of growth with continuous use over many years.

with seizures that are well controlled on **anticonvulsants** and are not of concern.

While side effects can be bothersome, none of them should become a reason for stopping a medication that is effective. Follow-up of side effects should be part of any medication trial and treatment program that attempts to treat ADHD symptoms to optimize functioning. It is your responsibility to report any untoward reactions that you experience to your treating physician and work with him on finding ways to reduce any side effects that do occur.

47. Do stimulants have a negative impact on blood pressure, heart rate, and/or other cardiac conditions?

Studies have documented that stimulant medications may cause a slight increase in average **heart rate** (about 3 to 6 beats per minute) or **blood pressure (BP)**. These increases are the average change seen in group studies, and some individuals, of course, may have greater increases. While these small changes would not be expected to cause problems in and of themselves, it is advisable that all patients taking stimulant medications for the treatment of ADHD be monitored for more significant changes in heart rate or blood pressure. In addition, greater caution should be exercised if someone who is considering stimulant medication to treat her ADHD symptoms has an underlying medical condition such as high or borderline high blood pressure or any other cardiac conditions such as heart failure, arrhythmias, or a recent heart attack that could lead to a life-threatening complication.

As a result of possible complications and reports of a few cases of sudden death in both adults and children taking stimulants at the usual dose used to treat ADHD, an FDA advisory panel urged that a black box warning be placed on all stimulant medications. This warning is meant to raise awareness in both physicians and patients and to foster additional caution. Therefore, it is of great importance that all patients (children, adolescents, and adults) have an evaluation of their cardiovascular status prior to beginning treatment with stimulant medication. This assessment should include two major components—a thorough discussion of medical history (both personal and family) for **structural cardiac defects**, fainting, **arrhythmias**, and unexplained sudden death; and a physical examination to ascertain the presence of cardiac disease. Further cardiac evaluation (including an **electrocardiogram** and/or an **echocardiogram**) is recommended if findings suggest any structural cardiac defects.

Sudden deaths have been reported in children and adolescents with structural heart defects taking the usual dose of stimulants. Stimulants should not be used in children with known structural cardiac defects or other serious cardiac problems. Likewise, because heart attacks, strokes, and sudden death have been reported in adults taking the usual dose of stimulant medication, doctors should only prescribe stimulants after a careful and thorough medical evaluation. Adults with ADHD who have coexisting cardiac abnormalities, coronary artery disease, heart rhythm abnormalities, or other serious cardiac disease should not be treated with stimulants. In addition, anyone who develops chest pain, fainting, or other symptoms suggestive of having a cardiac etiology while taking stimulants should be referred for an immediate cardiac evaluation.

48. When are stimulant (or nonstimulant) medications not recommended?

In addition to the cardiac restrictions for both stimulants and nonstimulants discussed in the previous questions, stimulants are not recommended for several other conditions. We will discuss the major ones next.

Pregnancy

Stimulants should only be used in cases where the benefit to the mother outweighs any risk to the fetus. (See Question 41 for a more in-depth discussion of pregnancy and ADHD.)

Glaucoma

Problems related to glaucoma may occur if blood pressure increases while one is on a stimulant.

Tics/Tourette's Syndrome

The association of Tourette's syndrome and ADHD is common.

The association of **Tourette's syndrome** and ADHD is common. For many years, it was believed that stimulants increased tics. However, several studies have not found this to be the case. Even at high doses, tics may stay the same, increase slightly, and then return to baseline levels, or they may even decrease on stimulants. The combination of clonidine and a stimulant (such as methylphenidate) have been found to be a safe and effective treatment for patients who suffer from both disorders.

Severe Anxiety or Agitation

Stimulants may increase anxiety and agitation; if you exhibit anxiety and agitation, you should avoid all stimulants, even coffee and caffeinated beverages unless your other symptoms are under control.

Mania

Stimulants may precipitate **mania** in undiagnosed or uncontrolled bipolar patients.

Bipolar Disorder—Untreated or Uncontrolled

You should not take stimulants if you have bipolar disorder unless it has been stabilized and is well-controlled. At that time, you might be prescribed very low doses of stimulants as an addition to therapy to reduce the symptoms of ADHD. However, as with all such conditions, you should be carefully monitored.

Preexisting Psychosis

If you are prepsychotic or have preexisting psychotic episodes, you should not take stimulants. Stimulants may precipitate frank psychosis. In stimulant overdoses, psychosis may be one of the symptoms seen.

Uncontrolled Seizures

For years it was thought that stimulants lowered the seizure threshold and might result in seizures. This too, has been questioned and is no longer thought to be the case. A low dose of stimulants has not been known to cause breakthrough seizures for those whose seizure disorder has been under control with anticonvulsants for many years. However, if you have uncontrolled seizures, you should not take stimulants for fear of increasing or prolonging the seizures.

Be sure to discuss any medical or mental health condition with your physician and provide him or her with a list of all medications that you are currently taking. Your physician will need this information to weigh the risks and benefits of treatment and discuss the appropriate use of stimulants to treat your ADHD.

Stimulants may precipitate mania in undiagnosed or uncontrolled bipolar patients.

Treatment of ADHD in Girls and Women

49. What is cognitive behavioral therapy, and when should it or psychotherapy and/or family counseling be added to medication therapy?

Cognitive behavioral therapies (CBTs) have recently been introduced to address the broad range of issues including self-esteem, relationship and family issues, daily health habits, stress level, and life management skills seen in adults with ADHD. CBT has been shown to effectively treat these ADHD-related issues particularly where medication alone has either little effect or takes a great deal of time to make a difference in the life of a woman with ADHD. In general, CBT challenges the ingrained negative patterns of thinking in women and girls with ADHD and encourages alternative scripts that reassure the woman or girl with ADHD that the outcome of events in her life are under her control and that she can make positive changes. Positive statements like, "I'm good in math," or "People like me when I smile!" can go a long way to helping a girl make academic progress or new friendships.

Neurocognitive psychotherapy, family counseling, and social skills training also provide tools that may be needed to address additional issues for girls with ADHD. Girls with ADHD often have great difficulty making and keeping friends and may benefit from therapy that focuses on developing social skills as well as boosting self-esteem. Adolescent girls with ADHD may need family sessions to work on oppositional behaviors (see Question 28 for a more in-depth discussion of the toxic mother/daughter dyad), problem-solving skills, and maintaining positive lines of communication among family members. In addition, they may need individual sessions to deal with individual stressors. Women with ADHD, as discussed earlier, typically develop a chronic sense of being a failure and are unable to meet the demands of daily life, leading to low self-esteem and chronic low levels of depression, issues that may need to be addressed through CBT and/or individual psychotherapy sessions.

In addition, other interventions often referred to as "neurocognitive psychotherapies" that combine cognitive behavior therapy with cognitive rehabilitation techniques proposed by both Drs. Nadeau and Young are proving quite effective for dealing with the day-to-day challenges that women with ADHD must face. Combining cognitive behavioral therapy that focuses on the psychological issues of ADHD (e.g., self-esteem, self-acceptance, self-blame, etc.) with the cognitive rehabilitation approach that focuses on life management skills for improving cognitive functions, learning compensatory strategies, and restructuring the environment has been found to be extremely effective when treating women with ADHD. As Ramsay and Rostain describe in their article, "Adapting Psychotherapy to Meet the Needs of Adults with Attention-Deficit/Hyperactivity Disorder," adults with ADHD who complete adequate treatment appear to have gone through a transformation in which ". . . patients start as disempowered 'victims' of ADHD, then become 'proactive' patients with ADHD, and, ultimately, leave treatment as individuals 'living' with ADHD, having integrated self-awareness and coping skills into their individual lifestyles" (Ramsay & Rostain, 2005, p. 81).

50. Is it true that meditation/yoga or a similar activity can actually be an effective treatment for ADHD?

Meditation and **yoga** can certainly be effective ways to improve focus and concentration, as well as provide a means to reduce stress caused by ADHD, but I would not go so far as to say that they are treatments for ADHD. Let's briefly discuss each one.

Yoga

Yoga combines stretching, physical movement, postures, and breathing with concentration and relaxation to help you feel more in control. Yoga requires a quiet space, usually indoors, but can be performed outside if you wish. It is another way to gain control over your body and develop deep relaxation. In addition, alternative therapies that incorporate a component of yoga, or are similar to the practice of yoga, reveal positive results in the therapeutic treatment of ADHD in children. One such method is meditation.

Meditation

Meditation has been used for years to help individuals improve their focus by concentrating on one thing (usually their breathing). Through meditation, you can learn to live in the moment and develop a more peaceful, calm state. Meditation is known to reduce blood pressure and pulse rates and to help people have a more positive outlook. Brief meditation techniques can also be used to help you refocus in the moment or as an on-the-spot stress reliever. The three-breath technique and mindfulness meditation are examples of such techniques.

The three-breath technique can be used to help you refocus and to reduce stress. The three-breath technique is quite simple. Just close your eyes and notice your next three breaths. As you do this, try to notice what else is going on around you, the sounds, the way your breath feels, the temperature or air on your skin, and so forth. As you do so you will notice a sense of well-being coming over you. In addition to this brief three-breath technique, another called "mindfulness meditation" can also be used to help you perform each and every act with greater attention in the moment. To find out if it is for you, try it for a while. Most libraries or bookstore have tapes/books on these meditation techniques. You can also look for a therapist or coach in your area who uses it as part of his or her practice. Mindfulness meditation can be difficult to learn, but it can be done practically anywhere and can improve focus and concentration.

51. Are there alternative therapies that I can try (e.g., herbs, nutrition therapy, behavior management, exercise, etc.) that have been proven to help ADHD?

Entire books have been written on this topic. To answer this question, I will merely be able to summarize some of the most relevant findings and point out which treatments entertain some promise for treating the symptoms of ADHD. **Alternative therapies** are usually defined as treatments other than medication and behavioral interventions (psychosocial intervention) that claim to treat the symptoms of ADHD with an equally or more effective outcome. These typically include elimination diets, supplements, working memory training, biofeedback, and other forms of training the brain, mainly with exercises.

Treatment of ADHD in Girls and Women

Elimination Diets

With elimination diets for ADHD, parents try eliminating certain foods from their child's diet to reduce ADHD symptoms. Over the past few decades, there has been much controversy about sugar, additives, food colorings, and preservatives and their relationship to ADHD symptoms such as hyperactivity. At this time, there is no proof that a diet high in sugar actually causes ADHD. Years ago, Dr. Benjamin Feingold, an adult allergist, offered the Feingold diet, in which he proposed the elimination of artificial colorings, flavorings, and preservatives in order to decrease hyperactivity in children. While many studies have disproved Feingold's theory, individual children who have tried this specific elimination diet have reported significant improvements. Some experts have proposed, however, that it is not the elimination diet, but rather the increased focus on the child that provides improved behaviors. A more recent study by McCann et al., published in 2007 in The Lancet caused the United Kingdom's Food Standards Agency to suggest that certain artificial colors, when paired with sodium benzoate, may be linked to hyperactive behavior.

Adding Supplements

Zinc

Some studies suggest that children with ADHD may have lower levels of zinc in their bodies. Improved symptoms, such as reduced hyperactivity and impulsivity, have also be reported in children with ADHD who took zinc supplements along with traditional ADHD treatment. A 2005 study published in the *Journal of Child and Adolescent Psychopharmacology* did show a correlation between zinc levels and teacher and parent ratings of inattention in children (Arnold & DiSilvestro, 2005).

Fish Oil

There is some evidence that fish oil can help improve ADHD symptoms. Fish oil contains omega-3 fatty acids. There are some findings that suggest that in children with ADHD who are 8 to 12 years old, fish oil supplementation may improve mental skills. For instance, it may help improve a child's ability to organize activities. In one study, a specific supplement of fish oil and evening primrose oil was used (Johnson et al., 2009). Results showed that it improved hyperactivity, inattentiveness, ability to think clearly, and overall behavior in children with ADHD who were 7 to 12 years old.

St. John's Wort

St. John's Wort is a common herbal supplement. It is used mainly for treating depression, anxiety, and sleep disorders. This herbal treatment affects brain chemicals, including serotonin, dopamine, and norepinephrine. Recent scientific studies do not support the use of St. John's Wort to treat ADHD. In fact, recent findings conclude that St. John's Wort has no effect on the symptoms of ADHD.

Brain Training

Neurofeedback

Neurofeedback intervention is based on findings that people with ADHD have a particular brain wave pattern. Neurofeedback treatment involves teaching the patient how to increase her arousal levels by changing this brain wave pattern. The patient's brain activity is monitored through electrodes hooked up to her head. When the brain waves reach a desired frequency, a signal informs the patient. Through training, the patient can ultimately learn how to increase arousal on her own. While there has been some promising research in this area, more research is needed to determine the efficacy of neurofeedback on ADHD symptoms.

Working Memory Training

Working memory is the ability to hold information in one's mind for later use and is important for attention and learning. This skill is important for recall of information on tests and other related tasks. Research has shown that children and adults with ADHD frequently have problems with working memory as well as other executive functions. Training programs, such as Cogmed Working Memory Training (www.cogmed.com), that can be done at home with the support and supervision of a trained coach have recently been developed and seem to demonstrate promising results.

Cerebellar Exercises

Cerebellar exercises are designed to develop the neural pathways and address the slow information processing and coordination deficits associated with ADHD. Through a series of physical exercises that combine movement and balance, these treatments are touted to speed up information processing and improve cerebellar functioning and ADHD symptoms. To date, these approaches have not yet been proven in a scientific manner to prove their efficacy in treating the symptoms of ADHD.

Cassie speaks:

I am always in search of ways to "cure" my ADD, from vitamins to medication. I know that a healthy diet and exercise, for me, is a prescription that helps tremendously. Medication and vitamins also help improve symptoms . . . somewhat. These things help mostly with my mood and keep me from getting depressed about my shortcomings.

There is so much talk about executive functions and how the brain can be trained and improve with games. Is there any research that this type of training can improve ADD? I have signed on to take a basic training course (40 sessions), and after that I plan to take the ADHD course to see if any of it helps my ADHD.

52. What else can I do to improve my ADHD symptoms?

Exercise! We have always known that physical exercise is important for our bodies, but we now know that it is also important for our minds. It can improve mood, give us energy, and change the levels of important neurochemical transmitters regulating pathways that are involved in ADHD. Dr. John Ratey has been writing about this for years and even has a book, *Spark: The Revolutionary New Science of Exercise and the Brain,* published in 2008 that discusses this important link. In it, he states, "To keep our brains at peak performance, our bodies need to work hard" (p. 4). So get out there and get moving!

Aerobic exercise can help people with ADHD reduce stress and better deal with their lives. The problem is that most people think that they need to join a gym, get on fancy exercise equipment, or work out in a 60-minute aerobics class to qualify. Well, that does not need to be the case. It can mean two 15-minute walks with your pet or 30 minutes of gardening. The struggle becomes how to motivate yourself to exercise *regularly.* Most adults with ADHD are turned off by boring or unstimulating exercise routines—I know that getting on that treadmill with nothing else to do is pure *torture* for me.

Aerobic exercise can help people with ADHD reduce stress and better deal with their lives.

Over the years, I have found that two important rules can help here—variety and brevity. Keep it short and sweet and add variety and spontaneity! According to the experts, even 20 to 30 minutes a day of physical exercise can provide substantial health (physical and mental) benefits. To motivate yourself, try the following methods:

1. *Join or create a group.* Join a mall walking group, schedule time each day to walk with a friend or join a team (rowing, soccer, basketball, even bowling). The company and commitment will keep you coming back.

2. *Get someone else involved.* Hire a trainer. Believe me, this will keep you motivated and on track. Once you see the results and hopefully get bitten by the exercise bug, you will be ready to go it on your own.

3. *Get a dog.* You cannot stay sitting down in front of the TV in the den when you have a dog—even in bad weather, pets need exercise! And they do a great job of reminding you of their needs!

4. *If you must walk on a treadmill, try to keep it interesting.* You can listen to music or watch TV, but I have found that if I watch a DVD of a movie I really want to see, I have a difficult time stopping, and cannot wait to come back the next day and the day after that until the movie is finished. Renting a 2-hour (or longer) movie gets you through four or five exercise sessions. I also find that DVDs of a TV series can keep you coming back for days . . . especially those HBO headliners like *Sex in the City* or *The Sopranos* . . . and each episode is timed perfectly for a great workout!

5. *Set a goal.* It might be as simple as walking around the block without huffing and puffing or walking (running) in a charity event next fall.

6. *Keep it simple and be creative.* Workouts of 10 minutes several times a day can add up. Try the old tricks of walking to the bus stop or parking farther away from the entrance to the mall. Garden, jump rope, or arrange to take the baby next door for a ride in a carriage! Her mother will love the few minutes alone or with her older children and you will feel better for it.

7. *Take the stairs.* I once knew a cardiologist who exercised by walking up and down the stairs of his office building several times a day between patients. Who says you are too busy?

8. *Get outdoors.* It has been well understood for many years that exposure to nature, measured by the number of plants in a home, the amount of nature (grass and trees) viewed from the windows of the home, and whether the home is surrounded by grass may protect the psychological well-being of children (and adults) and improve their attention and focus. Children with ADHD were found to concentrate better after a walk in the park. Just imagine what spending some more time outside can do for you!

PART FOUR

Other Issues

How do I break the cycle of inertia/procrastination
that has developed as a result of my ADHD?

How can I explain my ADHD and maintain
a positive relationship with my supervisor at work?

Why do women with ADHD seem to frequently
marry the wrong person?

More . . .

53. How do support groups or psychotherapy groups help women and girls with ADHD?

Meeting with others who have similar experiences can be both validating and empowering. Hearing the struggles and successes of other women with ADHD can provide insight into your difficulties and offer models for how you can deal with similar issues. Just being in a room where everyone else knows about ADHD and has experienced it firsthand can be extremely exhilarating. In the day-to-day world, that is often not the case, and a woman or girl with ADHD must live and work in environments where she may be the only one with the disorder. That can be a lonely situation!

A **support group** may be an informal get-together of people with ADHD or it may be organized and led by someone (either a layperson or professional) with knowledge of and interest in ADHD. While some support groups for parents have an affiliation with an ADHD organization like Children and Adults with ADHD (CHADD), others may spring into existence spontaneously. Adult groups may be affiliated with an organization or an ADHD clinic or private practice and have a professional leader or a mental health consultant, who merely observes and supervises. Other adult groups may consist of adults with ADHD, who have just found each other and banded together for support. **Psychotherapy groups** are somewhat different in that they are usually led by one or two professionals who either set an agenda or direct the discussion.

If you are unable to find a support group near you, think about starting one for local women with ADHD. The following are some tips for starting a support group from *ADDvance Magazine* (Vol. 1, No. 2, 1997, p. 27).

Tips for Starting a Support Group

1. Create a promotional piece to build interest in your group. Be sure to list a contact person.

2. Send your promotional material to targeted audiences (e.g., CHADD or ADDA, which is the National Attention Deficit Disorder Association) meetings, women's centers, social and religious agencies; arrange for public service announcements on local radio, TV, etc.

3. Use already established channels to collect information on interested women or mothers and daughters with ADHD.

4. Plan the initial meeting. Send out a notification of the time and place by e-mail, chat groups, posters, flyers, etc. (Be sure you have scheduled your meeting at a convenient time and place.)

5. Develop general guidelines for the group.

6. Remember, it will be exciting, but be sure you lead the group. Try to have an agenda for the first meeting and don't let things get out of hand or too off track. These are women with ADHD, so you will have to work hard to stick to the schedule or planned agenda.

7. Continue to promote your group and maintain contact with existing members.

8. Be attuned to members who might need extra support. Extra phone attention or referrals may be in order.

9. Be prepared for the group to change and to take on a life of its own.

10. Be prepared to stick with it even if things don't go as planned. You will be glad you did!

Other Issues

54. What special challenges do women with ADHD face, and what tools and techniques can help them meet those challenges?

The following is a list of various areas where ADHD symptoms seem to present a great deal of difficulty for women and girls with ADHD. Over the next several pages, we will explore each one in greater depth and I will offer tips and strategies for gaining control over these extremely challenging areas.

- Time management
- Organizationational skills
- Workplace issues
- Social skills issues
- Stress
- Hormones
- Relationships
- Motherhood and caregiving
- Parenting
- Sleep
- Athletics
- School

TIME MANAGEMENT

55. How do I break the cycle of inertia/procrastination that has developed as a result of my ADHD?

If you are like the majority of women with ADHD, procrastination is often a fixture in your life. Poor organization and time-management skills, difficulty planning ahead, all conspire to make it extremely difficulty for you to get work done in advance of any deadlines (even ones that you set for yourself!). Despite the best of intentions, time after time, distractions or unforeseen delays (like forgetting to get all the materials ahead of time) pop up and hold you back. However, with a little bit of insight and the proper planning you will be able to overcome that inertia and gain control of procrastination—even to the point of making it work for you!

Before you get started on developing a plan for dealing with procrastination, you will want to take a few steps to ensure the success of that plan. First, you will need to accept the fact that you are a procrastinator, and, second, gain a better sense of why you procrastinate. You will also want to analyze which symptoms of ADHD get in your way the most and investigate whether your medication helps you with those symptoms. If you observe that your medication does help you, make a mental note (or maybe write a "Take medication" sticky note to yourself) to be sure that you take your medication when you have work to do. Next, let's take a good hard look at the reasons why you procrastinate.

Reasons You Procrastinate

Before you get started on developing a plan, first, try to uncover some of the reasons for your procrastination. Ask yourself the following questions. Be honest with your answers!

- Do you have a poor sense of the passage of time?
- Does time simply "get away from you?"
- Do you have trouble estimating time?
- Do you find that you consistently do not plan enough time to complete a project before the deadline?
- Do you procrastinate in order to get the stimulation provided by being under the gun to get a project done on time?
- Do you enjoy doing things at the last minute?

- Do you like to live in the now and put everything else out of your mind unless it is right in front of you and needs to be worked on immediately or is due the next day?
- Do you have trouble determining what is the most important thing you should be doing right now?

If you have answered "yes" to many of these questions, you might be thinking, "Is there any hope for me?" The answer is, "Yes," but you will need to accept yourself and want to change. Let's get started on developing a plan for you to deal with procrastination.

Develop a Plan

Now that you are more self-aware, it's time to develop a plan that you think will work for you. The following are several options, choose one or try all three, to see what works best for you.

1. *Prioritize.* Start by analyzing and breaking down the project or task into its various parts. Next, look at what is the most important (or difficult) aspect of the task for you and then determine what you need to do to get *that* done. If you work on this part first, rather than leaving it for last, you will be more likely to get the entire project accomplished. Schedule a time to work on this specific part of the project. Make sure you write it in your planner or on your calendar or master schedule. Be sure to stick to your plan!

2. *Divide and conquer.* If a large project or a long-term assignment simply overwhelms you because it seems to be too much for you to possibly get done, causing you to do nothing until the last minute, try the divide-and-conquer plan. By breaking the task

down into smaller sections with individual due dates, you should be able to complete each task and thus the whole project on a realistic schedule, ahead of any due date. Just make sure to get the big picture and lay out your plans on a large visible calendar or white board. The bigger the better, so that the plan and due dates are difficult to miss. You might even use different colored pens to call attention to certain dates.

3. *Plan to procrastinate.* If you do decide that it works best for you if you wait until the last minute to work on a project, go right ahead, but PLAN for it. No guilt or added stress! Just accept that this is who you are and that you *can* work this way! If you need to use the momentum of working at the last minute on a project—plan for it! Get all the materials ahead of time. Set aside a time and a place and let everybody know your deadline and that you will be working nonstop until the project is finished. Ask that they not disturb you. Shut off the phone and computer and any other distractions. Once you are ready, go for it! Be sure to keep track of time. I will bet without the guilt and the stress, things will go much smoother.

56. Why is it so difficult for me as a woman with ADHD to be on time?

Managing time can be particularly difficult for a woman with ADHD. With the many competing demands for your time, it is easy to get off track and overwhelmed. In addition, it has been observed that it is difficult for many people with ADHD to judge the passage of time. I often tell women that, if you have ADHD, you most likely have only two concepts of time—now and not now.

For many women with ADHD, the first step in managing time is realizing that they can't. Instead of focusing on getting things done in a certain time frame or arriving at a certain time, it is better for them to just focus on getting the task done or getting there. Period. In my family, one of my sisters with ADHD was always late to family gatherings. We found that if she was bringing the appetizers for the dinner or party, we would all be waiting for her and getting hungrier by the minute. By the time she arrived, everyone was angry and upset. So, we decided to accept that she was always going to be late and not focus on it. For the next party, we assigned her the desserts. That way we could begin the party and enjoy seeing her whenever she arrived. And without the pressure, she always arrived well before dessert!

The second most common reason for not being able to be on time seems to be overcommitment. Taking on one more task (e.g., putting in a load of laundry) or running another errand (stopping at the dry cleaners and the pharmacy on the way to work) can ruin the best-designed morning schedule, and then you find you are late again!

Most importantly, however, you need to realize that chronic lateness is not just an irritant to you and others, it can have significant consequences. Tardiness can impact your relationship with others, jeopardizing your marriage, your friendships, and even your employment. I have worked with many, very competent women, who have lost their jobs because they were always late.

If it has become critical or you simply want to work on your ability to be on time, I recommend that you try the following strategies:

1. **Identify what gets you off track in the first place**. If you find that your problem is the passage of time, wear a watch with an alarm or set up visual reminders (schedules) of what you should be doing and when. If you are distractible, use that to your advantage. Post visual reminders (e.g., signs, sticky notes, or screen savers) in your environment to keep you to a schedule or to remind yourself to stay on track.

2. **Be accountable to someone else**. Make arrangements with a friend or coworker for phone or text check-ins to ensure that you are working on what you should be doing or leaving when you need to in order to be on time.

3. **Make a list**. If you tend to take on too many tasks in the morning, make a list of your morning routine and *stick to it!* Do not allow yourself to add one more thing!

4. **Hire a coach**! Working with a coach empowers many women with ADHD and provides the accountability and structure they need to follow through with their plans.

Rita speaks:

I wish so that I could be more on time. Even if I arise earlier, I still find little things to do, and time goes by at lightening speed. It annoys my husband, sister, mother, friends, etc. It comes across as rude, they say, and I really am a most sensitive and intuitive woman. I hate the thought of being rude, especially to my loved ones. This really is a constant burden. Also I am a night owl and find it difficult to wake up in the morning, but I force myself to get out of bed. It bothers me that my time clock isn't on the world's time clock!

Other Issues

ORGANIZATIONAL SKILLS

57. How does a woman with ADHD deal with (and explain to others) the confusion of being so focused and organized at times and distractible and unproductive at others?

In reality, the most consistent aspect of having ADHD is its inconsistency. The vulnerable ADHD brain is under constant bombardment from various stimuli from both your inner and outer environments and will function differently day-to-day or minute-to-minute depending on many factors. Attention and focus are dependent on both your motivation and the task—and the amount of stimulation or reward it provides. The boring nature of a task combined with the many steps that it takes to complete it (take laundry as an example—collecting, sorting, washing, drying, folding, and putting away) can make completing a task almost impossible. Hormonal fluctuations and irritating sensory stimuli can worsen ADHD symptoms, as well as mood and irritability levels in women with ADHD. (**Premenstrual syndrome [PMS]** has been found to be a particular problem for older girls and women with ADHD.) Lack of sleep can also wreak havoc with attention and memory after only one night of deprivation. Taking all these variables into consideration, it is no wonder your performance is so unpredictable. But how can a girl or woman with ADHD explain all of this to others without sounding like she is making excuses?

Hormonal fluctuations and irritating sensory stimuli can worsen ADHD symptoms, as well as mood and irritability levels in women with ADHD.

1. **Learn as much as you can about yourself**. Keep a diary or journal or simply jot down a few notes at the end of the day. Look for patterns and try to find links to other events or turmoil that may be going on. When do you do well and when is it harder to keep things together? Does your functioning

deteriorate as your medication is wearing off? Are things worse on the weekends when you do not take your medication? Are your ADHD symptoms worse right before your period? Do you find it more difficult to wake up or work in the morning? Do certain situations make you anxious?

2. **Share this information** with those who love and care about you. That way everyone will be on the same page. Knowledge can help you better understand how your ADHD is affecting you. However, keep in mind that your ADHD is an explanation of what is going on and not an excuse for bad behavior or poor performance. You will need to keep trying and do all you can to keep your ADHD symptoms under control. This means taking your medication as prescribed and taking good care of yourself.

3. **Make a plan** to keep disruptions, anxiety, and stress to a minimum. They all can make it more difficult for you to concentrate and stay on track. If worry and anxiety is keeping you from functioning at your best, be sure to discuss your feelings with your therapist or a trusted friend or advisor.

4. **Forgive yourself**. You and those around you need to realize that things are not always going to be perfect and that each day will bring ups and downs, but that you are trying and that is all that matters.

5. **Seek professional help** if you find that things are not getting any better, the medications you take for your ADHD do not seem to be working, or if your research reveals a more serious condition that needs to be treated such as anxiety, depression, PMS, or sleep disorders like obstructive sleep apnea or restless legs syndrome (RLS), all of which can further impair your functioning.

Keep in mind that your ADHD is an explanation of what is going on and not an excuse for bad behavior or poor performance.

Other Issues

58. Why do some women and girls with ADHD become perfectionists or develop obsessive-compulsive behaviors?

In an attempt to cope with their ADHD symptoms and the anxiety these symptoms generate, many girls and women with ADHD develop various compensatory strategies or coping behaviors. Some girls and women will blame others for their mistakes. Some may withdraw or let things go. But many women and girls, in order to deal with the anxiety created by symptoms that seem to sneak up and ambush them, will attempt to gain some semblance of control by becoming perfectionists. They make lists and check and recheck that their work is complete or that they have not forgotten important items before leaving the house each morning. Some may even develop strange habits or rituals. I remember one young girl who was brought in to see me because she was always lining up her shoes along one wall of her room. If they were out of order, she could not go to sleep at night without finding them all and lining them up where they belonged. As opposed to those with true **obsessive-compulsive disorder (OCD),** when asked, she had no compulsions and could provide a good reason for her seemingly bizarre behavior. It seems that in the past, she was always losing her shoes and could not readily find them in the morning before school. This problem had made her late for school on more than one occasion and she was very embarrassed by having to come in once the class had started. She vowed to do something about it to prevent it from happening again and lining up her shoes was her solution!

Some women with ADHD may also develop an **obsessive-compulsive personality disorder (OCPD)** in addition to their ADHD. These women may develop a preoccupation with details, rules, lists, order, organization, and schedules; exhibiting a perfectionism that interferes with many aspects of their lives. In addition, they may have difficulty completing projects or homework or take an excessive amount of time to get things right, never being quite satisfied. While some perfectionist or compulsive behaviors serve their purpose, these behaviors can also become overwhelming and create additional anxiety for girls and women with ADHD. If behaviors become too time consuming or rigid, the girl or woman may only be adding to her problems. She may only be able to concentrate on one area at a time (like the young girl's focus on her shoes) causing other areas in her life (e.g., social or personal) to suffer. In such cases, a therapist may need to be consulted to aid her in changing obsessions into healthier, more productive behaviors.

59. I always seem to have unfinished projects. How does this behavior go along with a diagnosis of ADHD and what can I do about it?

Unfinished projects are simply the result of your core ADHD symptoms. Difficulty with attention, distractibility, organization, and time management all contribute to unfinished projects when you have ADHD. If there is too much happening at one time, a woman with ADHD will often become distracted, lose sight of her goal, and feel frustrated at the end of a given time period because she can not see any visible results. At this point, she will be more likely to give up or move on to another project to have the same thing happen again as that project also ends up unfinished. She may also get stuck because of the way she organizes (or rather fails to organize) her things. Endless clutter mingled with supplies, books, stacks of paper, unpaid bills, unopened mail, used coffee cups, and various unfinished projects make it difficult to finish anything because having everything all mixed together makes it difficult to visualize what the finished project should look like. Don't despair! Here are several simple steps that will help you to deal with this issue.

First, you might want to take a look at the space where you work. Redesigning your workspace to better organize and accommodate your crafts and/or school or office supplies may allow you to be more efficient and accomplish more. Where you work is also important. Working in an office without a door or sharing an office or dorm room with one or more people, may be part of the problem. Retiring to a quieter space like an empty conference room, the library, a room without windows, or the basement of your home rather than the kitchen or family room with all the hubbub swirling around you, may be all that you need to finish a task.

Next, think about whittling larger projects down to a more manageable size. By dividing a project up into small chunks and tackling them one at a time, you will be less likely to give up as you see progress. Working in short chunks of time and taking frequent, short breaks may also increase your endurance. Another helpful tool involves making up target phrases that will get you back on task and help keep you there. These target phrases will help you maintain focus and increase staying power. Simple phrases such as "Focus!" or "Back to work!"

or "Almost done!" will help you stick to your projects until they are finished.

60. What are the pros and cons of paper versus electronic planning systems?

No organizing system is perfect, and most choices for using a certain planner or organizer are dependent on the needs of the person using them. If they are not designed to meet your needs or are not convenient to use, you will not use them, period! So, let's look at the pros and cons of both a paper and an electronic system and let you choose which one you think will work best for you.

Finding a Planner That Works Is the First Step
Planner Pads/Paper Calendars

Pros	Cons
Great for scheduling appointments	Not as good for daily schedules
Lightweight; easier to carry around	Easily lost
Pockets and folders added for bills, papers, etc.	Cannot organize e-mails, documents
	Need another space for a to-do list

Electronic Organizers/Computer Planners

Pros	Cons
Can be set up on a computer desktop	User needs to be computer savvy
Difficult to lose	Need backup file or system

Other Issues

Pros	Cons
User can set up as many desktop folders as needed	User may not be able to find folders
Holds all documents, e-mails, bills, etc.	Need online bill payment
Sync automatically with other people	
Sync with electronic to-do list	
Use time features to stay on task	

In the end, it is up to you. Which system do you think will help you the most? Which system do will think you will use! At some point you may want to try them both. Just be sure that you know how your brain processes information best and then choose a system that complements your own internal filing system.

61. How can I overcome a lifelong propensity to not put away my things?

Many women with ADHD live with a constantly cluttered environment, and with ADHD, clutter only tends to multiply! If you have not sorted through yesterday's mail, you are more likely to just toss today's mail on top of the pile and let the pile grow. There are no easy answers, but here are a few ADHD-friendly rules:

• *First, stop new clutter!* Before you tackle existing clutter, start by creating no new clutter. Hang up your clothes, sort and process your mail as it arrives, put things back after using them, put groceries on the shelves, fold the laundry and put it away, wash the dishes and put them away. Sound like a lot? It is if you try to do it all at once. Be kind to yourself and tackle only as much as you can handle. Try to focus on one area per day (keeping the sink empty and shined) and having it stay that way for a week or so is more manageable than keeping the entire kitchen or house clean. Have you ever heard of the Fly Lady (www.flylady.com)? She and her Web site are wonderful resources. She recommends starting with your sink and keeping it clean and shining. Soon, you will find that you are always putting the dishes in the dishwasher rather than in the sink, and everything just follows from there!

- *Think small.* Do not take on too much at once. Take on the sink or one drawer or shelf per day and then reward yourself for your accomplishment.
- *Finish what you start.* Take on one small organizing project at a time and then stick with it to completion. Make it enjoyable! Add a music CD or your favorite TV show and you have a half-hour or hour chunk of time to help you focus and stick to a task. Match boring tasks to ones that you enjoy. Folding laundry or exercising while watching TV makes the task less onerous.
- *Don't try to do it alone.* You or your family members and friends can work on this together. Ask your friends for ideas that might help with your clutter; ask them for support in digging out your rooms. I know one group of women with ADHD who visit each others' homes to help with laundry or cleaning tasks. They support each other in a noncritical way and provide the incentive to get the task done! Understand that being organized with ADHD does not come naturally, but with help you can do it.

(Adapted with permission from Quinn, P. O., & Nadeau, K. G. 2006. *When Moms and Kids Have ADD*, (expanded version), Washington, DC: Advantage Books, p. 62.)

62. How can I better handle tasks like boring housework versus activities I like to do?

If you are like most women with ADHD, the boring nature of most household tasks combined with the many steps that it takes to complete each one makes performing such tasks almost impossible. The following are a few tips that might help.

Do it first! Try doing the boring task first with the reward of doing something more enjoyable when it is finished. This reward-yourself strategy can provide the incentive you need to keep going until a task is completed. You can also make any task a little less boring by making it fun! Add loud music and dance as you dust, or watch TV as you fold clothes!

Pair it! You might also try pairing a boring task with another task that also needs to get done. A boring task refers to any task that is repetitive or that you have to leave and come back to, like laundry. With such tasks you will more likely to forget some of the steps or even that you were doing the task at all. What can you do to help with such tasks? Let's stick with doing the laundry as an example, since so many women with ADHD complain about getting it all done. First, pick a specific time each day when you can set aside time for laundry and another important chore that needs to get done daily as well, for example, going over your planner for that day or the following day. College students can review notes. Homeowners can pay bills. Just be conscious that you are doing laundry and (fill in the blank). Keep at it until you have finished both tasks. You will find that pairing these activities makes you more efficient. Depending on the second task, you can possibly even sit by the washer or dryer until the cycle is done. If you stay in the vicinity, you will be less likely to forget what you are doing! Just think—no more piles of dirty clothes or overdue bills!

Do it with a friend. Invite a friend who has the same problem, to keep you company and then reverse the process and offer to stay with her while she completes her boring task. The companionship will make the tasks more enjoyable and the time will go more quickly. You will also be there to keep each other on track.

Simply and eliminate. Probably one of the most effective ways of dealing with boring tasks is to eliminate as many as possible or at least decrease the number of times you need to repeat them. You can do this by creating a more ADHD-friendly household. *Simplify* and eliminate what you don't need. You would be amazed by what you can live without and how paring down makes life more manageable. Look around. Would bare floors be easier to maintain than all those rugs that need to be vacuumed? What about a house with fewer rooms? Open doors on closets and add hooks, pegs, and clear boxes to hold your belongings. Get the kids to help! Kids can dust! Pay them or hire help. Remember, a housekeeper is cheaper than a divorce or a breakdown! Get a job that you enjoy in order to be able to pay someone to do the tasks you don't.

> *Invite a friend who has the same problem, to keep you company and then reverse the process and offer to stay with her while she completes her boring task.*

> Simplify *and eliminate what you don't need.*

WORKPLACE ISSUES

63. Is it wise to tell my boss or colleagues about my ADHD?

Disclosing that you have ADHD may not always be the best decision in the workplace given the lack of understanding and knowledge about ADHD, especially in adults. I would recommend that you take a more cautious approach and consider disclosure only

Other Issues

when you have more information about how the news will be received. I have known many adults, who, once they disclosed that they had ADHD, found themselves under closer scrutiny and the target of even greater documentation and discrimination. But do not despair, there are alternatives to disclosure. In most cases, you do not need to disclose your ADHD in order to ask for accommodations. Rather than describing your ADHD in terms of a disability and demanding accommodations that you feel you are entitled to under the law, you might just as easily characterize it as a problem that you are having with a certain aspect of your work and then offer possible solutions. In this way, you will likely be viewed in a more positive light—as an employee who is trying to become more efficient at work and seeking support to accomplish that goal.

That being said, however, experts in this area like Dr. Kathleen Nadeau in her book, *ADD in the Workplace: Choices, Changes, and Challenges* (1997), point out that there may be circumstances under which disclosing your ADHD is warranted. First, you might consider disclosing your ADHD diagnosis to your coworkers if you feel that it (and you) would be met by a supportive reaction. You would be surprised by the number of coworkers who have relatives with ADHD who will be willing to help you accomplish your goals in the workplace. Second, you should consider disclosing your ADHD to your immediate supervisor if all other avenues have been exhausted and you fear losing your job if you do not get the help you need to get the work done. Finally, you should disclose your ADHD when you are in danger of losing your job because of poor performance. Disclosure may at least buy you some time to look into other jobs or to change the direction of your career. Reassessment of your diagnosis and the effectiveness of your treatment program should also be looked into at the same time. Minor adjustments in your medications may make you more productive and efficient, thus improving your performance. In addition, you should seek the help of a professional career counselor in order to better understand your strengths and weaknesses and career choices.

64. How can I explain my ADHD and maintain a positive relationship with my supervisor at work?

First, it is important that you have a clear picture of your ADHD, your strengths and weaknesses, and how they affect your performance in the workplace. You need to do this before you can set up a working relationship with your supervisor. You may even decide that you are best not disclosing your ADHD until you have established your supervisor's willingness to work with you (see Question 64 for a more in-depth discussion of disclosing in the workplace). Remember, it is up to you to help your supervisor understand you and your needs. You need to teach him or her how to work with you most effectively. Your supervisor and you have the same goal—getting the job done. If you start out in the relationship by acknowledging this mutual goal and then presenting ways you think you could better accomplish that goal, your supervisor will see you as a valued employee, not as someone defining herself by her ADHD.

Once you have established a working relationship with your supervisor, there are several steps that you can take to maintain the relationship. First, it is important to always remain positive. Remember, ADHD is an explanation not an excuse. Complaining and making excuses will do more harm than good. Make sure that you do not

It is important that you have a clear picture of your ADHD, your strengths and weaknesses, and how they affect your performance in the workplace.

only present problems, but that you offer solutions at the same time. For example, if you need regular meetings to keep on track with projects, do not begin by complaining about why you can not get things done, but instead, ask to set up these meetings and explain how they would help you meet your deadlines. Be sure that you are reasonable with your requests. You can not expect your supervisor to be available at all times. Asking for a brief, regularly scheduled meeting is often most effective and easier to accommodate. Working together toward meeting your goals, will make success in the workplace more likely, and nothing will ensure a more positive relationship with your supervisor than your success.

65. What strategies can I use in the workplace to minimize the negative effects of my ADHD?

Symptoms such as inattention, inability to sit for long periods of time, impulsivity, poor attention to detail, and distractibility can all affect women in the workplace as well as at home. By using strategies that address specific issues, you can improve your functioning in the workplace without specifically disclosing your ADHD. The following are just a few you might try.

Minimize interruptions. To minimize interruptions and noise in the work environment, ask to work in an empty conference room or office, or wear headphones designed to reduce ambient noise. You might try coming in earlier or staying later than your coworkers to give yourself some extra quiet time when fewer people are around.

Move It. It is also important to look for opportunities to move around as much as possible. Exercising during a lunch break can refocus a sagging **attention span**

and has been proven to decrease restlessness and hyperactivity. Likewise, the need to fidget during meetings can be assuaged by doodling, taking notes, or fingering an object like a pen or paper clip.

Use reminders and routines. To improve punctuality or to stay on track, set an alarm on a watch or computer to provide a cue for changing tasks or as a reminder to go to a meeting. Setting up a routine time (daily or weekly) to report to your supervisor can be another important way to stay focused and on track with projects and assignments.

Learn to say "No." Women with ADHD often have difficulty saying "no" when asked to do a task resulting in their taking on too much, which leads to increased stress and pressure. To avoid being overscheduled, always check your calendar before committing to a new project, to make sure that you have time to fit it in, and do not give in to the impulse to do one more thing!

Stick to a schedule. In many jobs, it is also easy to get sidetracked by various tasks like answering e-mails or overwhelmed when working on multiple projects. To better deal with all these distractions, it is important to set limits. Each day, set aside a specific time to answer e-mails or work on a specific task; put it on your schedule and stick to it. Let your coworkers know your schedule and when they can expect a response. Set a timer on your desk or on the computer to keep you on track and to remind you when it is time to move on to other tasks. Folders on the computer can also be set up to keep projects and tasks separate. Keep everything labeled and on your desktop. Placing items randomly in the My Documents folder may result in their being lost forever!

Other Issues

Setting up a routine time (daily or weekly) to report to your supervisor can be another important way to stay focused and on track with projects and assignments.

Placing items randomly in the My Documents folder may result in their being lost forever.

Ask for help. Finally, ask for help when you need it. If you are not good at filing, ask someone who is skilled at it to help you organize your files, but make sure that the system you set up *works* for you. If you have problems with writing reports or composing memos, have someone help you set up some standard outlines that you can use for various projects. Keep the originals in an appropriately labeled file folder on your computer. When you need to generate a document, you can pull up the outline and add a few sentences under each section. This technique works well for fax covers, routine reports, standard memos, invoices, expense reports, or any document that you need to generate on a regular basis. I have used it in my practice and other businesses for years and have found it makes me more efficient and better able to get reports or evaluation results out in a more timely fashion.

Susan speaks:

My name is Susan and I'm a 47-year-old, who works as an office manager for a real estate firm. I have had four major jobs in my 31 years of work life. Everyone thinks I'm such a strong person and a go-get-'em type personality. . . . However, as a little girl, I could never finish projects on time and often stayed up late at night crying and frustrated that my little sister (6 years younger) could finish her homework, but I couldn't. My mother would help me, but later lost interest and told me to finish myself or fail—my choice. This scenario lasted all 12 years I was in school. No, my mother never took me to a doctor to find out the reason for my slowness.

Throughout my school years, I considered myself a failure. I could not finish schoolwork and my mother would get mad at me for not completing my household chores. She often called me Cinderella dreaming someday my prince will come. I never really thought of the part of dreaming. I think most of my life I dreamed of things to come, doesn't everyone? My mother would say that I daydreamed most of the time and that I would play with my dolls in my room for hours. When my mother would talk to my siblings and me about serious issues or chores, or whatever, I would daydream and leave the conversation (going somewhere in my mind) and she would then tell me to "Stay with everyone," or ask me "Are you still with us? Hello in there."

Now as an adult, I've noticed that I cannot focus on my daily list of projects to complete. I have good intentions to complete them; however, I never seem to have time to accomplish them. I get easily distracted, literally start refocusing, then some other project pops into my brain and I stop and move to that project. I work 12 hours a day to feel ahead of the game so tomorrow I'm not as backlogged. I work over the weekends to get ahead on next week's projects (that were really this week's projects). Coworkers e-mail me, telling me they told me something last week; why can't I remember? Or they send me an e-mail, I answer and then they would send another. At that time, I feel overwhelmed by so many e-mails and multiple conversations. I can't keep up with so much information. When I type at work or send a simple e-mail, you should see what comes out of my brain—all misspelled words, words ahead of other words. I need help or someone to tell me I'm not crazy or lazy! What can I do? I'm afraid I'll lose my job!

66. Are certain careers more ADHD-friendly than others?

While some careers may require certain qualifications that make them more uniquely suited for individuals with ADHD, in general, it is not the particular career

Other Issues

that is important, but rather how well-suited the person with ADHD is for that career. When looking into a career or considering available job options, it is important to understand your unique skills and strengths and try to make the best match possible. These include your interests, accomplishments, personality, and work habits, as well as the special challenges that ADHD present for you. In addition to books on the subject, such as, *Finding a Career That Works for You* by Wilma Fellman, a career counselor can also assist you in the process of finding the best career match. The suggestions that follow will help get you started.

To begin the process, make a list of the qualifications, as well as any specific advantages and disadvantages, of each career that you are considering.

To begin the process, make a list of the qualifications, as well as any specific advantages and disadvantages, of each career that you are considering. Next, make a separate list of your unique strengths, weakness, and qualifications. Then compare the two lists. By looking at them together, you should begin to see which career fields and jobs best match your skills. For example, if you note that you have strong people skills and poor organization skills, you should only look at those jobs that match your strong people skills (e.g., flight attendant or salesperson), and avoid ones that require organizational skills (e.g., administrative assistant or accountant).

Certain jobs and careers, however, are innately more ADHD-friendly than others. An ADHD-friendly job, as described by Dr. Kathleen Nadeau, is one that can provide some or all of the following characteristics:

- Tasks that are usually assigned according to an employee's strengths
- Support
- Flexibility
- Encouragement
- Regular communication with management

- Constructive problem solving
- Minimal paperwork
- Structure and routines
- Flexible work styles—teamwork versus solo
- Autonomy with guidelines and backup support
- Long-term projects that are divided into defined, short-term tasks with real deadlines
- Opportunities for creativity and individual input. (Source: Nadeau, K. (1997). *ADD in the Workplace: Choices, Changes, and Challenges*. New York, NY: Taylor and Francis Group.)

For individuals with ADHD who tend to get bored easily, a job with greater inherent stimulation (like emergency room work and other related careers such as an emergency medical technician (EMT), fire fighting, or police work) can make all the difference. In addition, people with ADHD should seek out careers that offer a great deal of variety with minimal paperwork. Some adults with ADHD have discovered that they are able to satisfy this need by working two part-time jobs rather than a full-time job or by remaining in "the field" rather than accepting a promotion to a boring desk job. Last, remember, that when you are pursuing your passions, work never really seems like work!

Melanie speaks:

My name is Melanie, I am 27, and I have been diagnosed ADHD for 1 year. Unfortunately, in my profession there is a lack of support and to a certain point a lot of ignorance about disabilities like ADHD. At the moment, I'm working as an event coordinator. I have found that my disability affects me at work in the following ways:

- *I can't manage to stay focused on the tasks, because I work in an open space with people coming and going all day long.*

- *I tend to make mistakes when handling and presenting data and Excel worksheets, such as budgets or matching guest lists.*
- *I struggle to finish the projects within the deadlines.*
- *I always seem to have a never-ending list of unfinished tasks.*

The owner of the company has given me 6 months to change this pattern, otherwise I must go. Nevertheless, my supervisor is very supportive and has asked me what she can do to help me to cope with the challenges of this job. I don't know which type of job I should be looking for that would go with the flow of my ADHD symptoms: flexible hours, possibility to delegate work, having assistants, and being able to choose projects? I may need to change jobs soon!

SOCIAL SKILLS ISSUES

67. How does ADHD affect social skills in girls, and what can parents do about it?

Girls with ADHD often have problems making and keeping friends. A girl with inattentive subtype ADHD may be shy and withdrawn, making it more difficult for her to join groups or to speak to someone she does not already know. Lack of attention to visual cues or body language can make reading other girls' intentions difficult. As a result of these social skills deficits, a girl with ADHD may sit on the sidelines and have problems joining a group that is already engaged in an activity. Girls with combined subtype ADHD have opposite problems. They may be hypertalkative, monopolizing the conversation and not giving others a chance to speak. They may be bossy or always changing the rules of games, causing others girls to reject them. However, they may also be unaware of others' reactions to them and miss social cues.

How Parents Can Help

One way to help your daughter with ADHD build friendships is by focusing on her relationships with *one* or *two* children at a time. This goal can be accomplished by arranging supervised, time-limited, playdates so that your daughter can spend time with another child to practice her social skills. Make sure that the playdate has an organized activity and that you are there to supervise. By inviting your child's friend to a *highly* attractive activity—for instance, the movies, bowling, or an amusement park, the invitation is more likely to be accepted. Be sure to review social goals with your child *prior* to these social activities. Go over what will be expected of her and role-play various scenarios so that she will be better prepared and feel more comfortable.

You can also help your daughter develop improved social awareness by spending some time together practicing how to read facial expressions or body language. You can do this by going to a park or playground together and observing other children playing in groups and pointing out and commenting on their behaviors. It is also fun to watch TV with the sound muted and try to guess what is going on by facial expressions and other behaviors.

You might also enlist other family members in the process so that your daughter can practice her newly acquired social skills. Cousins make good friends and playmates and sometimes have an advantage over siblings, who may be less cooperative. You might also involve your child's teacher and guidance counselors in helping to reinforce social skills at school. Some schools have social groups, sometimes called a "lunch bunch," hosted by the guidance counselor during lunchtime that focus on building social skills.

It is also important to remember that it is okay for your daughter to only have one or maybe two good friends. Your aim is not to have your daughter win a popularity contest, but to support her as she learns the important social skills that make relationships work. Also keep in mind that your daughter may feel more comfortable being friends with a boy that she knows well and plays with often than other girls. Friendships with other girls can be a lot of work, often requiring a great deal of attention to detail and sophisticated social interactions and language skills, making these friendships difficult for girls with ADHD.

68. What about a girl who is shy and withdrawn and has difficulty making friends and talking with others? How can she be helped?

As I discussed in the answer to Question 69, making and keeping friends can be a challenge for girls with ADHD. However, girls with ADHD can learn these complex social skills. There are several ways that you can help. In her book, *How to Raise Your Child's Social IQ*, Cathi Cohen states, "Practicing social skills is like practicing a musical instrument or a sport. Everyone needs to practice, but different levels of natural talent will require different levels of effort" (Cohen, 2000, p. 19). Some girls with ADHD will need more practice in this area than others. Cohen goes on to state that, "Often times, children need to role-play and then practice in a real-life situation, and then role-play again" (p. 19). It is the practice that actually gives girls with ADHD the confidence they need in social situations.

In providing opportunities for a girl with ADHD to make friends, it is important to first help her identify and pursue her interests. In these settings, she is more likely to find children with the same interest and have something in common to talk about right away. It is also important to increase social opportunities. Create time and space for her friends within your home. At first, you may want to limit the amount of time for these play-groups. Anticipate and rehearse these encounters and what will most likely be said (role-play), and make sure you familiarize your daughter with the afternoon's agenda. Assure her that you will control the situation, as best you can, and that there will be no surprises for her. Be sure you are available to supervise and observe the small group interactions (without interfering). After the play-time is over, you can go over what went right, and help your daughter achieve new skills by role-playing any interactions that were problematic, offering alternative behaviors and scripts so that your shy daughter will feel more confident and comfortable in these social situations. Remember, practice makes perfect!

69. What can be done if you are a woman who is always changing her mind or saying things she regrets?

One definition of **impulsivity** is acting *or speaking* without thinking. For a woman with ADHD, impulsivity may be the main reason for saying and doing things that she later regrets. But if this is part of her ADHD, how can she turn this situation around? One way is to figuratively put on the brakes. A woman who is always saying things she regrets needs to focus on slowing down! Counting to 10 in her head before she speaks, asking herself if she would give the same response if she were in front of a large audience at her church, or imagining a piece of duct tape across her mouth that she needs to remove before she speaks may all help her think *before* she speaks.

For a woman with ADHD, impulsivity may be the main reason for saying and doing things that she later regrets.

She might also step back and analyze when she is more likely to speak out and say something she regrets. Is it when she is off her medications, or late in the day when she is tired? Do certain people encourage her to misbehave or say and do things that she later regrets? Avoiding these manipulators and their negative influence may help her regain control. Waiting 10 minutes before she makes a decision or sleeping on it and making a decision in the morning are additional ways that can slow down impulsive decisions.

70. How does one deal with the swirl of thoughts and overcommunication associated with ADHD including interrupting, being too loud, or starting completely different conversations, and so forth?

The communication problems listed in this question are all significant issues when a woman has ADHD, so let's attempt to tackle them one-by-one. Impulsivity and distractibility can cause one to jump into a conversation at the wrong time or start talking about completely unrelated topics during conversations. I have often been known to finish a conversation I started several days before whenever it pops into my head. So, how does someone with ADHD avoid sending the wrong message and stop from saying too much or jumping in at the wrong time? Let's develop some visuals and prompts to help with these problems as we did in the last question.

I have often heard impulsivity described as having no filters. Whatever comes into your head comes out of your mouth. To address overcommunicating, I would suggest trying to visualize something like a filter or tape across your lips or that your lips are "locked" and you need to go get the "key" before you speak. Both techniques should slow you down enough to ask yourself if the person you are speaking with really wants to hear what you are about to say or if it is appropriate.

Second, try to make *listening* and not *speaking* a priority by really focusing on not interrupting. Once you are aware that you have a tendency to not listen and rather think about what you are going to say, you might visualize a stop sign or a giant ear as prompts to slow yourself down and better focus on listening. You might also try thinking about a conversation as a game of catch. Only the person with the ball can speak. Therefore, you cannot speak until the other person finishes and throws you the ball. Then it is your turn. If you think you might forget what you are going to say, start carrying around a small notebook or keep paper by the telephone and jot down notes to help you remember what you want to say. If this is not possible and the thought is really important, you might briefly interrupt the person speaking, but be sure to apologize and explain that you have something important to say and that you fear you will forget. Ask the other person to remind you to tell him about it later when he finishes speaking. That way you really have not interrupted or changed the conversation and you have conveyed that you feel that what the other person was saying was important.

Try to make listening and not speaking a priority by really focusing on not interrupting.

Third, consider medication for ADHD and whether it might help you with these important communication areas as well. Medication for ADHD can effectively decrease distractibility and impulsivity and may help you slow down enough to focus on what is being said. If you take medication, see if you notice improvements in these areas while your medication is working. Try to pay attention to how long your medication actually lasts and if you find you interrupt more or are louder

Medication for ADHD can effectively decrease distractibility and impulsivity and may help you slow down enough to focus on what is being said.

Other Issues

when it wears off. You may need to have a discussion with your healthcare provider about taking a longer-acting medication or taking your medication on weekends to help you better address these social skills issues.

Don't be afraid to ask for help if you need it.

Last, don't be afraid to ask for help if you need it. Let others know that you are aware that you have problems in certain areas of communication and share that you want to work on them. Ask them to gently let you know if you are interrupting or talking too much. It may help them (and you) to know that you value their friendship and that you are not doing these things on purpose. By explaining how your ADHD sometimes makes it impossible for you to keep still, you are not making an excuse, but sharing that you want to change.

STRESS

71. Does stress affect ADHD?

As stress increases, ADHD symptoms tend to increase as well.

As stress increases, ADHD symptoms tend to increase as well. Symptoms such as short attention span, disorganization, forgetfulness, and poor management of daily tasks are often magnified by stress. But the reverse is also true. When you reduce stress in your life, your ADHD becomes more manageable. So, how do you reduce your stress levels? It is not always easy, but the following steps might help.

It is important that you learn to recognize the signs that you are becoming stressed.

First, whether you are a girl or woman with ADHD, it is important that you learn to recognize the signs that you are becoming stressed. These signs might include increased irritability; headache or stomachache; feeling that your heart is pounding; tight muscles in your jaw, neck, or shoulders; or problems sleeping. Next, try to find out what is causing your stress. Conduct a **stress analysis** and make a list of the things that cause stress in your daily life. Then use this list as a guide for reducing stress. Identify situations or people who are particularly stressful or toxic for you. Try to avoid the situations that cause you the most stress like running late in the morning, forgetting important papers or books, or having an argument. Since all situations and certain people cannot be avoided, you should also learn to use one or two of the more common stress-management techniques. Common stress-management techniques include **deep breathing**, **progressive muscle relaxation**, aerobic exercise, and yoga. The benefits of exercise are discussed in Question 52 on page 95, so, lets briefly review the others here.

- *Deep breathing.* When someone or something has upset you and you feel angry or stressed, try deep breathing to help yourself calm down and get back in control. It's simple! Take a deep breath through your nose as you count to 10. Hold that breath for the count of 4; and, then let your breath out slowly through your pursed lips to the count of 10. Repeating these steps four or five times should make you feel calmer. The trick is to remember to use this technique when you get upset.
- *Progressive muscle relaxation.* Although this technique takes a bit longer and requires more practice, it is a wonderful way to relax and can actually help you settle down during the day or fall asleep at night. By tightening and relaxing the muscles in every part of your body, you can release stress and become calmer. Try this exercise when you get in bed. You can also do it lying on the floor or seated in a chair. Start by closing your eyes. You then tighten, hold for the count of 10, and release different muscle groups, starting with your toes and feet and progressing to your legs, buttocks, abdomen, chest,

arms, neck, and face. Remember, you are only tensing one muscle group at a time, and be sure to breathe slowly as you perform this exercise. When you finish, you should feel more relaxed and may even drift off to sleep.

- *Yoga.* Yoga combines stretching, postures, physical movement, and breathing along with relaxation and concentration to help you feel more relaxed and in control. Yoga practiced regularly has been shown to help with many of the symptoms of ADHD. For instance, children with ADHD who practice yoga demonstrate a decrease in hyperactivity and impulsivity, and an increase in attention span and self-esteem. In addition, alternative therapies that incorporate a component of yoga, meditation, or mindfulness meditation reveal positive results in the therapeutic treatment of ADHD in children and adults. (Yoga and meditation are also discussed in Question 50.)

Seeking Outside Help

If stress becomes overwhelming and/or it affects your health and overall well-being or your daughter's, it may be time for you or her to see a therapist or counselor to work on stress reduction. A therapist can work with you on identifying stressors that can be reduced and help you deal with them more effectively.

HORMONES

72. Do hormonal fluctuations affect ADHD symptoms in girls and women?

It has been proposed that whenever brain estrogen levels fall below the "minimum brain estrogen requirement," for whatever reason and at whatever age, brain functioning worsens. Low estrogen levels are particularly problematic for women and girls, who are already

A therapist can work with you on identifying stressors that can be reduced and help you deal with them more effectively.

experiencing ADHD symptoms as a result of a neuro-transmitter imbalance. Hormonal changes occurring at puberty can affect girls with ADHD, causing them to become emotionally hyperreactive. These girls, as well as women with ADHD, often tell me that they feel like they are on an emotional roller coaster. Low estrogen or widely fluctuating hormone levels may be the underlying cause of this emotional turmoil.

Low estrogen states occur prior to your menstrual period each month, after you have a baby, and during menopause, although hormone levels begin to decline several years before your menses actually stops. This latter stage is referred to as perimenopause and can begin up to 10 years before actual menopause. (See Question 73 for a more in-depth discussion of menopause and its effects on ADHD.) Symptoms shared by women in low-estrogen states include depression, irritability, sleep disturbance, anxiety, panic, difficulty concentrating, and memory and cognitive dysfunction. Women with ADHD frequently report a worsening of their ADHD symptoms during these low-estrogen states. In addition to worsening ADHD, each month, some women with ADHD report that they experience both the physical symptoms and the mildly depressed mood of PMS, or the more severe depression and other disturbances of **premenstrual dysphoric disorder (PMDD)**, which can significantly affect their ability to function.

Women with ADHD frequently report a worsening of their ADHD symptoms during these low-estrogen states.

73. *How is menopause likely to affect my ADHD symptoms?*

As you enter your late 40s and early 50s, it is important that you become aware of several perimenopausal and menopausal issues that affect women, but especially those with ADHD. First, menopause comes with a whole host of symptoms, including memory problems and mood changes, in addition to **hot flashes**, insomnia, and other physical symptoms experienced by many women. You might find that you have difficulty with short-term **verbal memory**, **word retrieval**, and mental clarity. These symptoms are now thought to result from the decreasing estrogen levels that can affect brain functioning. As a woman with ADHD entering menopause, you need to work with a physician who is aware of the interaction between ADHD symptoms and estrogen levels.

Perimenopause begins when estrogen levels start to decrease and occurs several years before actual menopause. It is a time often associated with mood changes and the onset of depression in some women who have had no previous history of the disorder. Perimenopausal women report feeling sad, irritable, tired, and worried, as well as having difficulty sleeping. This depression and the **cognitive deficits** associated with decreasing levels of estrogen that occur prior to and during menopause may cause a woman with ADHD to have greater difficulty coping with her ADHD symptoms as well. She may find herself becoming less functional with more severe ADHD symptoms as she enters this phase of her life. This is often the reason a woman will seek help for her ADHD for the first time in her late 30s, 40s, or early 50s. At that time, she may seek out a diagnosis from a physician because she can not longer cope with her worsening symptoms. If she has been diagnosed previously and is receiving treatment for her ADHD, her medications may not seem as effective as her symptoms worsen with menopause, and the dosage may need to be adjusted at this time.

Your physician needs to take all of this information into account and design a holistic approach to assist you in getting back on a more even keel. It may take some trial-and-error to find what works for you, because no two women have the same needs. You might need an increase in your stimulant medication, and you will likely need symptom coverage for 16 to 20 hours per day. In addition, any sleep issues you have need to be addressed. Your doctor should consider prescribing multiple doses and/or combinations of **short-acting stimulants** and **long-acting stimulants** to be taken along with a stimulant. **Antidepressants** and estrogen or **thyroid hormone** replacement may be warranted if other serious conditions such as depression or hypothyroidism coexist with your ADHD.

You should also make it a habit to practice good self-care during these stress-filled phases of your life. Good self-care includes eating a wholesome, nutritious, well-balanced diet and getting plenty of exercise and sleep. Discuss your symptoms with your physician and bring up the possibility of other treatment options including **vitamin supplements**, omega-3 fatty acids, alternative therapies, and possible hormone replacement therapy to boost estrogen levels. Above all, be kind to yourself and get all the help and support you can to make this difficult transition time more comfortable.

Laura speaks:

I was diagnosed with ADHD a year ago. It was a relief to know that something was different about the way I lived, processed information, and why I seemed oblivious to some things, yet very focused on others, etc. I went on medication (Adderall XR) and felt brand new, almost driven to complete tasks that I quickly burned out on before taking medication. Now, some days, it seems the medication doesn't work as well as before, and some days, I wonder if I even remembered to take my pill. I'm noticing the muddled feeling that I had noticed before I started medication creeping back in, even on medication. My physician has increased the dose of my medication but these problems continue. I have noticed some hormonal changes as well. I started on oral contraceptives to try to even out my hormones, with the help of Celexa. Both have helped me with the severe PMS I was experiencing, but not these other symptoms. I am 47, almost 48 now, and feel that my decreasing hormone levels are affecting my ADHD and its treatment.

RELATIONSHIPS

74. How can ADHD affect sexual intimacy?

While the effects of ADHD on marriage and social relationships have been studied and discussed for some time, little attention has been focused on the issue of how ADHD affects **sexual intimacy**. Yet, more than any other social area, intimate relationships are likely to be affected by deficits associated with ADHD. In intimate relationships, you must be wholly present in the moment and attentive to responses within your own body as well as to the other person. You must be astute at reading subtle visual cues and body language to ascertain the likes and dislikes of your partner. Reading body language requires attention and focus and has long been a problem for women with ADHD. A woman's distractibility can often be misinterpreted as disinterest or result in behaviors that ruin the mood altogether. I vividly recall the story of one woman with ADHD, who, while engaging in foreplay with her husband, distractedly remembered that she had no milk for the children's breakfast in the morning. At once, she got out of bed, dressed and went to the store.

When she returned home she could not understand why her husband was so angry!

Sensory issues associated with ADHD (discussed in Question 31) may make light touch, stroking, or intimate physical contact uncomfortable. A tendency to rush may cause some women to want to skip foreplay altogether in order to "just do it." In addition, to achieve **orgasm**, a woman must be able to focus and concentrate on bodily sensations and be present in the moment. Noises or other distractions at that time may make it impossible for her to achieve climax. To improve focus and concentration, sex therapists have recommended that women with ADHD who experience problems in this area take their stimulant medication prior to having sex. By improving concentration, stimulants have allowed many of these women to achieve orgasm (some for the first time!). If a woman with ADHD seems to be having problems in these areas, I suggest that she see her physician or schedule an appointment with a sex therapist who knows about ADHD. She and her partner will be glad she did!

To achieve orgasm, a woman must be able to focus and concentrate on bodily sensations and be present in the moment.

75. Does ADHD affect dating behaviors?

Just as boredom and need for stimulation affect job satisfaction, these same factors can affect a woman's dating behaviors. Often women with ADHD do not recognize how their symptoms may affect almost every aspect of their lives, including dating. They go from relationship to relationship never stopping to analyze how ADHD may be contributing to the problems they experience. Irritability, emotional reactivity, and poor communication skills cannot help but negatively affect the quality of relationships. Impulsivity may cause a woman to say things she regrets or lead to one breakup after another. No wonder, women with ADHD express

Impulsivity may cause a woman to say things she regrets or lead to one breakup after another.

dissatisfaction in their relationships or give up on dating altogether.

Treatment for ADHD symptoms is critically important to maintaining or improving your dating/romantic relationships. I remember working with one young woman with ADHD who took forever to realize that she was constantly arguing with her boyfriend on the weekends when she did not take her medication. Once I pointed this out to her and she began taking her medication every day, their relationship became much smoother.

A woman's choice of dating partners may also be affected by her ADHD. Long-standing self-esteem issues may lead her to believe that she is not worthy and cause her to choose partners who are not a good match. Other women with ADHD break up repeatedly or fail to pursue dating relationships because they perceive that the prospective boyfriends are too good for them or not able to accept them with their problems and failures. Realizing that no one is perfect may help these women make better decisions or be willing to stay in relationships longer. Understanding that ADHD will not go away and that, as a couple, they and their partners must confront the daily toll that ADHD takes can be the first step to improving relationships. Seeking additional individual help or attending couple's therapy, if necessary, can provide additional support and understanding.

When to disclose her ADHD can also be a significant issue in the dating relationship. A woman should not disclose too early, but conversely she should not hide this important part of herself if a serious relationship has developed. In any relationship, timing is important.

Sari Solden, author of *Women with Attention Deficit Disorder,* cautions, "Just 'coming out' with a statement that you have ADD, when someone doesn't understand what that means might not be helpful." She further reminds women that they ". . . don't want to keep a secret for too long in a relationship either because then that itself can become the issue" (Solden, 1997, p. 12). In the beginning, a woman might just talk about her strengths and weaknesses, which would be natural in any relationship. As she feels more comfortable and both parties have lived with each other's vulnerabilities for awhile, revealing her ADHD will be easier as it is an essential part of who she is.

76. Why do women with ADHD seem to frequently marry the wrong person?

Choosing a spouse or partner is perhaps one of the most important decisions we will ever make. And yet, the decisions about whom we marry are often influenced by our attraction to the person we are with at the moment. However, these feelings can often obscure the facts that surround a lifelong commitment. Women with ADHD are prone to impulsive decisions, often not thinking through the consequences of marrying the wrong person.

Women with ADHD often choose to marry people who possess the qualities they lack. Whether they are aware of it or not, women with ADHD are often attracted to those who seem to fill in the deficits they perceive in themselves. Because of their poor organization and management skills, these women are drawn to others who possess these skills and who they think will keep them on track. This person, however, may turn out to be extremely controlling and difficult to satisfy. Thinking they have chosen an organized person, ADHD

Other Issues

Choosing a spouse or partner is perhaps one of the most important decisions we will ever make.

Women with ADHD often choose to marry people who possess the qualities they lack.

women marry, only to find that the marriage brings with it many demands that they are unable to fulfill, making their feelings of worthlessness and inadequacy even greater. When a spouse/partner is overly critical or controlling, marriage can be especially trying. Sometimes these marriages may work, if the partners complement each other and build a relationship that is based on each other's strengths.

Other women with ADHD may choose to marry someone who also has ADHD, feeling that because these men are just like them they will understand their mistakes and shortcomings. While the spontaneity of such relationships may be exciting at first, they can also lead to serious problems if ADHD symptoms are not held in check. With no one paying the bills, reining in spending, or taking care of household tasks, things can get out of hand pretty quickly. These relationships tend to work no better than controlling ones, often ending in finger-pointing, anger, and frustration. Rarely, however, when both individuals receive treatment for their ADHD and are aware of how ADHD affects each of them and their relationship, such a marriage can provide a wonderful, mutual support system.

What Can You Do?

First, *be aware of your values and needs!* Second, while dating, be on the *lookout for subtle clues*. How does your significant other make you feel? Empowered or down on yourself? Accepted and valued for your good qualities or ashamed of your weaknesses? Is your prospective spouse willing to learn about ADHD and be part of the solution rather than add to your problems? Instead of blaming and criticizing you, can you work together to resolve issues that occur in all relationships?

You should also *listen to others*. What are they saying about this person when you are dating? Are your friends and family telling you that your boyfriend/significant other is not right for you? Are they telling you there is a problem with the relationship or how you are handling it? Be open, listen carefully, and weigh what they are trying to tell you. They have an outsider's perspective, and your judgment may be clouded by your love, impulsivity, or other ADHD traits. Above all, is the person you are with willing to work on your relationship? Would he consider going with you to therapy to avoid conflicts or deal with other issues you may already have encountered in your relationship? If not, he may not be willing to stick around and work things out after you are married, either. All of this may sound like work, rather than romance, but all rewarding relationships take effort and commitment!

77. How does ADHD affect marriage?

Inattention, impulsivity, hyperactivity, and poor organizational skills can all significantly impact the social life of an individual with ADHD, but can wreak havoc in a marriage. As a result of these ADHD symptoms and the stresses they create, a high percentage of marriages where one partner has ADHD end in divorce. Many couples are unaware of ADHD and the role it plays in their marriage. But that does not need to be the case. Knowing about ADHD and how it can negatively impact your relationship, however, can help you address these issues before the situation deteriorates to animosity or even more devastating situations for all involved.

Let's take a closer look at the symptoms of ADHD and see how they can affect a marriage when a woman has ADHD. In a traditional marriage, the wife is usually the person responsible for setting up the schedule and family appointments, keeping track of and caring for the kids, planning and preparing the meals, and keeping the clothes clean and available. If she is a woman with ADHD, tasks such as struggling with organization, time management, and staying on track may become almost impossible for her. As a result, she struggles constantly, often staying up late into the night, only to get further behind. Working outside of the home only adds to her stress. A woman with ADHD is often the true desperate housewife!

The negative situations created by her ADHD often lead to a downward spiral in the home and the relationship. Her husband will often have difficulty understanding why she can not seem to accomplish what other women can do. Her sloppy housekeeping skills may be interpreted as laziness or not caring. He may become frustrated and angry that his wife cannot meet his personal and emotional needs. She in turn feels inadequate that she cannot meet her husband's and her family's expectations. All becoming significant factors in the failure of her marriage.

Maria speaks:

I am a 44-year-old woman mother of three children. All three children and I have been diagnosed with ADHD (three out of four of us have ADD and my youngest son has ADHD and oppositional defiant disorder). The father of my children is the only member of our family who does not have ADHD. He asked for a divorce 5 months ago, and I am convinced that ADHD is a significant factor in the failure of our marriage. He blames me for the problems with the children and for my lack of attention to him and everyday household duties. Our divorce is extremely hostile. I stayed home 16 years to raise our children and their father is not willing to take into account our special needs in his view of our separation. He wants to sell the family house, which would force my children to change schools (I would not be able to relocate in the same area with my share of our community estate); and he wants custody of the children half of the week (which would remove a lot of stability and routine from their lives). He never really understood what it is to live with ADD or ADHD despite my many attempts to share books or articles on the subject with him.

78. What does it take to make a marriage work when a woman has ADHD?

In a successful marriage between a non-ADHD man and a woman with ADHD, understanding and negotiation are often the keys to success. Roles and responsibilities will often need to be negotiated based on each partner's strengths. By analyzing household responsibilities and ascertaining who is best suited for a task, rather than assigning tasks based on inflexible traditional roles, the disappointment and blame that follow when a job is not done can be avoided. Each spouse should take on the roles for which he or she is best suited and look for ways to minimize or eliminate problem areas. Asking, "Is this a good job for you or me, or should we look for someone outside of the family to fill this role?" is a great place to start. I often recommend the book, *A House-keeper Is Cheaper Than a Divorce,* by Kathleen Fitzgerald Sherman to women with ADHD. A husband would do better to ask what he can do to help rather than constantly criticizing, or complaining. This simple approach can go a long way in decreasing tensions and preventing hurt feelings within a marriage.

For a woman with ADHD, success in her marriage or in her family life depends in large part on setting up an ADHD-friendly environment with realistic expectations for herself and for her husband. Her level of self-knowledge and commitment to her treatment program will often be the critical factors that carry her through the day-to-day stress and challenges. By minimizing the negative aspects of ADHD, she will be way ahead in keeping her marriage intact. In addition, a woman with ADHD should do all that she can to educate her husband and family about her ADHD. Sharing books and pamphlets, visiting Web sites on ADHD, and attending meetings together will help foster understanding and help them clarify the role ADHD plays in their relationship.

Finally, a woman should not lose track of some of the positive aspects of ADHD. She should cherish her creativity and fun-loving spirit. Having fun together with her spouse whenever possible can dissipate the worst of moods and keep the spark alive in their marriage. She should save up positive memories and pictures from their early days together to draw on when things are not going as well. A sense of humor and not taking ADHD too seriously will help her and her husband and their marriage get through the toughest times.

79. How can I explain ADHD to my husband so he will understand my struggles and frustrations?

An ADHD-friendly marriage is one in which both spouses understand the impact of ADHD and work together to find solutions.

To create a more ADHD-friendly life, a woman with ADHD must work hard to educate all the people in her world about the impact ADHD has on her and about her efforts to take charge of these challenges. It is hard enough being a woman with ADHD without being surrounded by others who blame you for your difficulties! This is especially important when it comes to your spouse. An ADHD-friendly marriage is one in which both spouses understand the impact of ADHD and work together to find solutions. Information about ADHD, its symptoms, appropriate treatments, and strategies to reduce its impact can allow you and your husband to begin to work together toward a resolution of many issues and problems you face. It can also help your husband to let go of resentment and to accept that you are not acting deliberately. It gives you both hope that things can change!

ADHD, however, should never be used as an excuse. It is an explanation of why you may act in a certain way, but you still need to work with your husband to develop solutions to problems that you encounter on a day-to-day basis. Be open and honest with him about your symptoms and how they affect you, and express your willingness to seek treatment and work on a program to minimize your symptoms' intrusion in your marriage. By sharing your feelings and your eagerness to work together, your spouse will be less likely to feel alone in dealing with issues that arise in your life together. I have spoken with many couples whose marriage has ended in divorce because of undiagnosed or untreated ADHD in one spouse, who confess that they would still be married if the affected spouse had received treatment for ADHD during the marriage.

ADHD, however, should never be used as an excuse.

MOTHERHOOD AND CAREGIVING

80. How does ADHD affect parenting/caregiving?

Motherhood is a difficult role for which few of us are prepared. When you add ADHD to the mix, being a mother becomes even more challenging. Women are more likely than men to be the primary parent of their children, and women with ADHD possess the strong likelihood of having a child with ADHD. As the

Motherhood is a difficult role for which few of us are prepared.

abundant literature on children with ADHD attests, raising a child with this disorder is a particularly challenging task, made even more daunting when the mother has ADHD herself. And, when a marriage ends in divorce, it is the mother who is most likely to have custody of her children. All of these interrelated patterns strongly illustrate the potentially much greater challenge that parenthood poses for women with ADHD rather than for men.

Yet, while great attention has been paid to the parenting needs of children with ADHD, very little attention has been paid to the needs of mothers with ADHD and the ways that recommended parenting approaches must be adapted to their needs. One study found that mothers with ADHD who have children with ADHD were more likely to have relatives with alcoholism and other psychiatric disorders, more likely to have psychiatric disorders themselves, and more likely to experience problems with daily living compared to mothers without ADHD (Weinstein, 1998).

A more recent study published in the *Journal of Abnormal Psychology* provides the first data on how parents with ADHD perform on key parenting tasks (Murray & Johnston, 2006). Results from this study documented the parenting difficulties experienced by mothers with ADHD. Compared to other mothers, mothers with ADHD provided less supervision and were less knowledgeable about their children's whereabouts, friends, and activities; were less consistent in their discipline strategies; and generated less effective solutions to child-management problems. It is interesting to note that mothers with inattentive subtype ADHD (those with inattentive symptoms, but not hyperactive-impulsive symptoms) appeared to have greater difficulty with monitoring and consistency than moms with ADHD combined subtype. But it is not all bad news! Despite these difficulties, moms with ADHD were no less positive than other mothers in how they related to their child and provided their child with similar levels of positive feedback and support.

Colleen speaks:

I am a mother of three young children and I have ADHD as do two of my children. I find that in order to keep things running around our home, I sometimes hyperfocus in order to complete tasks. I was wondering if there had been any studies done on the children of ADHD mothers and how a mother's behaviors emotionally affect her children. I worry that when I tune them out in order to think, they feel less valuable. This breaks my heart, but, I must do this in order to keep up with all that has to be done. When I stop to look and listen to them, I lose track and momentum. Doesn't that sound terrible? I do try to set aside parts of the day when I can devote one-on-one attention with each child, but I find that this is not always enough. It takes so much of me to keep my home orderly and I worry that it seriously affects my children.

81. How can a mom with ADHD be most helpful to a child with ADHD when both are struggling with similar issues?

When a mother has ADHD, her first step should be to get treatment for her own ADHD issues. Instead, a mother's usual tendency is to focus on her child's difficulties while neglecting her own. Just as a passenger on an airplane is told to put on his or her own oxygen mask before assisting his or her child, a woman with ADHD must first get help for her own ADHD before she can effectively deal with her child's problems.

When a mother has ADHD, her first step should be to get treatment for her own ADHD issues.

A mother's usual tendency is to focus on her child's difficulties while neglecting her own.

Other Issues

By talking to her child about her struggles, a mother can begin the process of positive change for both herself and her child. By taking the steps to gain control over her ADHD, a mother helps both herself and her child. In addition, she becomes a positive role model. Her child will be able to see that with the right kind of help, he too, can function better at home and at school, just like his mom.

ADHD should be viewed as a family affair.

Second, ADHD should be viewed as a family affair. The reality is that everyone is affected when several family members have ADHD, and all need to work together to create an environment in which each family member can feel and function better. Instead of only focusing on a child's ADHD problem behaviors, it is important to find creative solutions that involve the entire family. Together, they will be able to tackle their ADHD challenges with humor and mutual support, leading to a better life for all members with and without ADHD.

An excellent tool to address issues and to foster change within a family is the **family meeting**. When everyone participates in finding solutions, each person is more likely to be motivated to change. Regular family meetings can create and reinforce feelings of acceptance and belonging. Family meetings are a time to discuss issues, plan activities, and practice problem solving. Whether meetings are held on a weeknight or weekend, be sure everyone can attend. Use this time to come together to focus on solutions, not problems; on progress, not imperfections. *Our Family Meeting Book: Fun and Easy Ways to Manage Time, Build Communication, and Share Responsibility Week by Week* by Elaine Hightower and Betsy Riley is a great resource to help you structure family meetings. This practical guide offers 52 simple agendas for weekly meetings that are fun and easy for everyone.

82. When a mom has ADHD, what is the best way for her to establish/maintain consistency and order in her family?

One mother with ADHD succinctly described this challenge by asking, "How am I supposed to organize my child when I can't even organize myself?" Daily life in many families when several members have ADHD can be chaotic. Developing daily routines, particularly a morning routine and an evening routine, can help your family become more orderly. Work on developing these routines as a family and be sure to problem solve as a family when a routine is not working. The following are some questions and suggestions to help your daily routines go more smoothly.

Developing daily routines, particularly a morning routine and an evening routine, can help your family become more orderly.

Setting up a Morning Routine

A morning routine begins with getting out of bed and ends with departing for the day's activities. Different family members may have different routines, but they all need to be coordinated. Before setting up a routine for your family, you will need to make a few decisions including:

- What time should each family member get up in the morning?
- What should be done if that family member over-sleeps?
- Who needs help getting ready for school and who will help them?
- What time is breakfast and who prepares it?
- When and how will each person depart?

Some suggestions that may help you problem solve when the morning routine is not working smoothly include:

- Maybe the late sleeper needs an earlier bedtime or a better alarm system.
- Maybe the can't-find-my-shoes kid needs to lay out clothes the night before.
- Maybe it would help to have healthy grab-and-go breakfasts available for mornings when someone is running late.

Setting up an Evening Routine

A successful morning routine depends upon a good evening routine. When you make preparations in the evening and get to sleep on time, your morning routine will go more smoothly. An evening routine should specify such things as:

- Homework time for each child.
- Bath time for each child.
- Preparations for the next day—making lunches, setting out clothes, and collecting items needed for school or work.
- Get-in-bed time for each child.
- Lights-out time for each child.
- Just as important, a go-to-sleep time for mom.

Many women with ADHD sabotage their own morning routines by staying up too late reading or watching TV. They then have difficulty getting up in time to supervise an organized morning routine for the children. (Adapted with permission from Quinn, P. O., & Nadeau, K. G. 2006. *When Moms and Kids Have ADD* (expanded version). Washington, DC: Advantage Books, pp. 39–40.)

83. How can a woman thrown into the role of caregiver for an elderly parent get everything done at home and keep from being overwhelmed?

To deal with these real-life situations, a woman with ADHD needs to look for creative solutions to specific issues related to the "sandwich generation" as she raises kids with and without ADHD. When you are a mother with ADHD it can seem impossible to get anything done. So, what can a mother with ADHD do when she needs to respond to multiple demands all competing for her time? It is never easy, but the following tips might help you use your time more efficiently:

- *Schedule early morning quiet time.* Onc mother with ADHD became an early bird, getting up at least an hour before the rest of the family. She described her morning time as her island of peace before the storm of the day. This hour was her time to plan, prioritize, and take care of any paperwork, such as insurance forms that needed to be mailed or permission slips that were being sent to school that day.
- *Go be a kid!* Another mother used the phrase, "Go be a kid!" to let her children know it was time to go outside or into the family room and give her some uninterrupted time. It is important to have a safe place (a fenced yard area if your children are younger and want to play outside), where you can keep an eye on them without having them underfoot. While your children are busy being kids you will have time to make a few uninterrupted phone calls, make a grocery list, sort through the mail, or relax for a few precious minutes.
- *Schedule mom's quiet time.* Teach your kids that mom needs quiet time. Even young children can learn to

To deal with these real-life situations, a woman with ADHD needs to look for creative solutions.

When you are a mother with ADHD it can seem impossible to get anything done.

Other Issues

give you a few quiet, uninterrupted moments if you train them on a daily basis, rewarding each child who has not interrupted you during quiet time.

- *Schedule kids' quiet time.* Teach the kids that they need quiet time, too. Quiet time in their room engaging in a low-key, enjoyable activity is good for kids with ADHD and helps them decompress when they are overstimulated. Teaching kids about quiet time—both yours and theirs—is an important lesson in learning to live with ADHD.

- *Create a traveling desk.* Use a zippered, fabric shoulder bag to neatly store your checkbook, stamps, pens, address book, paper clips, felt-tip markers, etc. Within your traveling desk, keep a zip-closure, see-through plastic folder to store bills to be paid. (Zip closure is important so that nothing can fall out.) Keep another zip-closure folder for other paperwork. Then, when bills or other paperwork arrive in the mail, or when kids bring forms from school that need to be completed, store them in your traveling desk.

- *Use your lunch hour at work for home-management tasks.* Try doing personal paperwork at work during your lunch hour. Bring your traveling desk to work each day. Many women find that they have more energy in the middle of the day to pay bills, balance the checkbook, or write a letter than they have later in the evening.

- *Use waiting time to do paperwork.* If you are like many moms, you spend a big chunk of your week taking kids to lessons and sports practices. If you have your traveling desk with you, you can set up your office anywhere. Waiting time in doctor or dentist's offices is also a great opportunity to get paperwork done.

- *Tag team with your partner to free up some additional time.* If you have a spouse or significant other, who is a parent figure in your family, coordinate with him so that you can get some uninterrupted time away from the kids and other responsibilities to take care of tasks that require concentration.

- *Stick to* your *program.* Above all be sure to set aside some time each day to take care of your personal needs. Take medication for your ADHD as directed, and do not forget to get regular exercise and much-needed sleep. Skipping any of these important tools will make everything else much harder to accomplish. (Adapted with permission from Quinn, P. O., & Nadeau, K. G. 2006. *When Moms and Kids Have ADD*, (expanded version). Washington, DC: Advantage Books, pp. 47–49.)

84. The many tasks of mothering and constant kid distractions/demands bring out my ADHD symptoms more acutely and make me cranky and short-tempered. What can I do?

When the day is long, frustrations build, conflicts develop, and arguments between parent and child with ADHD can rapidly escalate from irritation to out-of-control yelling. Each reacts to the other, pouring fuel on the fire. Research suggests that mothers with ADHD who do not take medication for their ADHD to keep symptoms under control are particularly prone to arguments and corporal punishment. The following are some suggestions to minimize conflict and its aftermath.

First, make sure that your ADHD is under control and your medication is effective even at the end of the day. Try taking a few steps to make the evening go more smoothly. You might find that you feel more rested and less prone to irritation if you take 15 minutes of quiet

You might find that you feel more rested and less prone to irritation if you take 15 minutes of quiet time before trying to deal with all you need to do during the evening.

155

time before trying to deal with all you need to do during the evening.

Try to find time at the end of each day to be with your child in a loving way.

Second, try to find time at the end of each day to be with your child in a loving way. No matter how many conflicts you have had during the day, work hard to find a way to end the day on a better note with your child. Bedtime can be a special bonding time rather than another occasion for argument. Spending a few minutes together, reading or talking, after your child is in bed can provide calm after a frustrating day.

Third, try to analyze the patterns of your conflicts so that more can be avoided. Do you and your child seem to take out the day's frustrations on each other? When your child yells, is your reaction to yell even louder? Are your battles centered on homework? If so, perhaps it would work better if someone else became your child's homework partner; this could be the other parent, a tutor, or even an older teenager.

Last, make conflict-avoidance a joint project. Talk to your child about the arguments and yelling. Apologize for previous behaviors and make a decision to tackle your problems as a team rather than blaming your child. Try to pinpoint the times when arguments are most likely to happen. In many families, angry explosions are more likely around dinnertime when everyone feels tired and hungry. Would a healthy predinner snack help your child feel calmer? Could you and your child agree to separate and calm down before continuing a discussion that has turned into a fight? By doing all you can to keep things calm, you will not only feel more in control, but you will be setting a good example and modeling important problem-solving behaviors for your child(ren). It seems like a win-win situation!

PARENTING

85. What parenting style should I adopt if my daughter has ADHD? Disciplinarian? Compassionate mentor? Drillmaster? What is the best parenting style for a mother with ADHD to employ?

Both questions call for a discussion of parenting styles, so I will address them together in this answer. First, let's examine what the term **parenting style** means, how each style affects a girl with ADHD, and then turn our attention to parenting styles and mothers with ADHD. It is important to point out that parenting style is much broader than any specific behavior, like a mother who yells or ignores and fails to supervise her children. While these behaviors do influence a child's development, researchers have found that broader patterns of parenting have a greater effect on a child's development and success. The theory of parenting styles was initially developed by Diana Baumrind (1971). She initially proposed that parents' behaviors fall into one of three categories: **authoritarian parenting style** (practiced by parents who tell their children exactly what to do), **indulgent parenting style** (practiced by parents who allow their children to do whatever they wish), or **authoritative parenting style** (praticed by parents who provide rules and guidance without being overbearing). The theory was later extended to include **negligent parenting style** (practiced by parents who disregard the children and focus on other interests). Let's examine each of these parenting styles a little closer and see how they might affect a girl with ADHD or a woman with ADHD and her children with and without ADHD.

Parents who use an authoritarian parenting style are usually demanding and make most or all of the decisions for a child.

Parents who use an authoritarian parenting style are usually demanding and make most or all of the decisions for a child. They do not consider their child's preferences or allow the child to have choices, thus providing few opportunities for the child to learn from her mistakes. Communication between parent and child are usually limited to commands and subsequent punishments when expectations are not met. In addition, authoritarian parents may hold unrealistically high expectations for grades, without giving their child the assistance she needs to be successful. Although this approach leads to obedient behavior in the short-term, children reared in this way often report greater feelings of unhappiness, low self-esteem, and problems maintaining friendships. A girl with ADHD already experiences many failures in her life. The home should be a place of understanding and a safe environment where, with support from her parents, she can learn new skills. In addition, this type of parenting provides few opportunities for her to practice problem solving or to learn from her mistakes.

Indulgent parents usually adopt a more permissive parenting style. There is little structure or organization within the home and few stated behavioral expectations. A girl with ADHD within such a home may feel confused, never really knowing what is expected of her. As she desperately craves structure, she may even act out to get her parents' attention and feedback. Many permissive parents want to change and will typically set up some structure at one point or another. However, when their daughter pushes back, they renege and allow her to take control once again. Indulgent parenting thus results in a girl with ADHD who has difficulty regulating her own behaviors. Being accustomed to having her own way and lacking accountability, she may encounter problems with other forms of authority and not achieve academic success.

Authoritative parents are both demanding and responsive. They create and monitor clear standards for their daughter's conduct. Parenting behaviors are both assertive and supportive. They respond to their daughter's needs, taking her ADHD into consideration. Yet, these responses would be considered empowering rather than enabling. These parents are more open to a natural give and take with their daughter with ADHD. They foster self-advocacy by allowing her to express herself and encourage her to get her needs met. This style of parenting results in daughters with ADHD who are happy, competent, and academically successful.

Last, negligent or uninvolved parents provide only for their daughter's basic needs, but are not at all supportive or encouraging. They often fail to monitor and supervise her activities. These parents do not establish and reinforce long-term goals. A girl with ADHD raised by uninvolved parents would not learn many of the skills necessary to overcome her ADHD, and will be seen as lacking self-control and self-esteem. In addition, such girls may engage in risk-taking or out-of-control behaviors to get the attention they crave.

Parenting Style for a Mom with ADHD

Mothers with ADHD have a great deal of difficulty with organization, consistency, and providing the structure their children need, often making them look indulgent or permissive. When observed and compared to mothers without ADHD, moms with ADHD more often did not know their children's whereabouts. In addition, they lacked flexibility in problem-solving

Authoritative parents are both demanding and responsive.

Negligent or uninvolved parents provide only for their daughter's basic needs, but are not at all supportive or encouraging.

Other Issues

159

skills, causing them to have difficulty generating solutions to everyday problems. While these behaviors may cause them to also appear uninvolved, this seeming failure is more likely the result of their distractibility and lack of attention to what is going on. Their children may have told them where they were going, but they simply were not listening. To achieve a balance and incorporate a more desirable authoritative style, mothers with ADHD will need to espouse a two-pronged approach.

If you are a mom with ADHD, you can set up a program to become a better parent. First, you will need to get your own ADHD under control. Stimulant medication has been shown to not only improve ADHD symptoms, but can also reduce inconsistent parenting and decrease the use of corporal punishment. Medication dosages may need to be optimized, however, to provide coverage throughtout the day and well into the evenings and on the weekends.

Parenting programs are also essential for learning effective strategies and providing parenting tools.

Next, you will need help achieving a balance between meeting your own needs and those of your child(ren). Therapists, ADHD support group members, and coaches can help you develop a plan and stick to it. Having someone to talk to who knows what you are going through can make all the difference in handling parenting responsibilites more evenly and consistently. You will also more likely be able to stay on track if you can take a break from parenting to relax and recharge every once in awhile. Enlist the help of others (babysitters, house cleaners, grandparents, your spouse, older siblings, friends, etc.) to schedule regular daily or weekly breaks. Parenting programs are also essential for learning effective strategies and providing parenting tools.

However, these programs should be undertaken only after your symptoms are under control to gain the most benefit.

86. Is parent training effective if a parent has ADHD? Should I take a parenting course to help me be a better parent?

Despite the importance of this issue, there has been only limited attention to the topic of parent-training programs' effectiveness when the mother has ADHD. To date, there have been two studies that looked at ADHD symptoms in parents and related them to the effectiveness of parent training. In the first study of mothers with high levels of ADHD symptoms, it was found that their children with ADHD showed no improvement following parent training, while mothers with few ADHD symptoms had children who bene-fited strongly from this intervention (Sonuga-Barke, Daley, & Thompson, 2002).

In another study published in the *Journal of Attention Disorders*, the authors assessed parenting behavior in mothers and fathers (aged mid-20s to mid-50s) of chil-dren ages 4 to 12 years before and after taking parenting classes. In general, fathers who reported symptoms of inattention and impulsivity were found to be more per-missive and reactive before and after parenting classes. The degree of impulsivity reported by these fathers was also associated with more arguing with their children before parenting classes. Mothers with inattentive symp-toms were found to have lax parenting skills both before and after parent training. These results suggest that par-ent training programs are not as beneficial when a parent has untreated ADHD (Harvey et al., 2003).

Parent training programs are not as benefi-cial when a parent has untreated ADHD.

161

87. How can I start a family when I already have so many problems with my own ADHD?

I often hear this question from young women with ADHD. It is usually when they are struggling with their ADHD symptoms and see only the problems that they are having at the time and not the possibilities for when things get better and they are more in control. However, life rarely is so black-and-white, handing us such all-or-nothing choices.

Remember Nobody's Perfect

In dealing with your own ADHD, it's important to always consider yourself a work in progress and not seek perfection.

In dealing with your own ADHD, it is important to always consider yourself a work-in-progress and not seek perfection. If we all waited to be perfect before having children, the world would be vastly underpopulated! It is more important to be prepared than perfect! Once you are on medication and your treatment program seems to have you in a better place, you will be better prepared to make a decision about becoming a parent.

Prepare for Pregnancy and Newborn Parenting

It's more important to be prepared than perfect!

Once you have decided that the time is right (or you find that you are pregnant), it is important that you schedule an appointment with the physician who treats your ADHD as well as your obstetrician or family practitioner. At that time, you should discuss all medications you are taking including those for your ADHD (see Question 41 for a discussion of stimulant use during pregnancy), and any other conditions (e.g., antidepressants, anticonvulsants). Many of these medications can cause harm to the fetus and may need to be discontinued prior to or during pregnancy.

After the baby is born, your hormone levels will rapidly decrease. This relatively lower-estrogen state can wreak havoc with your ADHD. (See Question 72 for a discussion on low estrogen states.) You will also be getting less sleep. These factors make it critical that you take extra care to get lots of rest and decrease stress during this important time. ADHD symptoms are sure to worsen when you are sleep deprived or under stress. Ask for help when you need it and work on simplifying your life as much as possible. Newborns do not know that you have ADHD—they just need your love and attention.

Parenting Your Young Children

The most important thing to remember about parenting is that no one ever has it down completely. If you think you do, your child grows and develops, his needs change, and you will feel like you are back at square one! Remember, we all make mistakes. Look at your strengths, instead of only seeing the difficulties you experience. You are in a better position than mothers who took on the role of parenting before they knew they had ADHD. From where I stand, that looks like you are way ahead of the game!

You also need to remember that you are not alone. Join a support group like CHADD (Children and Adults with ADHD: www.CHADD.org) or the ADHD Moms community on Facebook (www.facebook.com/ADHD-Moms); attend parenting classes offered by local community groups, universities, or your church (make sure your ADHD symptoms are treated first). (See Question 86 for an in-depth discussion on how to get the most out of parenting classes); and read as much as you can. An excellent place to begin is with the book *When Moms and*

Take extra care to get lots of rest and decrease stress during this important time.

Ask for help when you need it and work on simplifying your life as much as possible.

Other Issues

Kids Have ADD written by Dr. Nadeau and myself. Be sure to check out the "Resources" section at the end of this book for more suggestions. You should also know that parenting is difficult for everyone, but that you also bring some very exciting qualities to the role. Mothers who have ADHD are often more empathetic and less critical of their children's failures and foibles, having experienced many themselves. In addition, many mothers with ADHD are extremely creative and have lots of fun with their kids! They design the best Halloween costumes and plan many fantastic backyard adventures and spontaneous good times! As one mother with ADHD recently shared with me, "I might not know what I'm doing with my kids, but I can guarantee it's going to be fun!"

SLEEP

88. How does ADHD affect sleep?

Women with ADHD often complain about having difficulty "shutting off" their brains at night to go to sleep.

Women with ADHD often complain about having difficulty "shutting off" their brains at night to go to sleep. They report that their thoughts jump around from one concern, thought, or worry to the next, resulting in significant difficulty with falling asleep (initiation insomnia). They report that once they finally fall asleep, their sleep is very restless. They toss and turn. They awaken to any noise in the house. In the morning they often find the bed torn apart and the covers kicked onto the floor. Most report that their sleep is not at all refreshing, resulting in excessive daytime sleepiness and fatigue.

Sleep disorders are very common in adults with ADHD.

ADHD and sleep disorders have not been the subject of a great deal of research, but the few studies that have been conducted, nevertheless, report that sleep disorders are very common in adults with ADHD. Adults with ADHD report going to bed later, have a wider range of bedtimes, were more likely to take over an hour to fall asleep, and were more likely to experience difficulty going to bed, going to sleep, sleeping restfully, or waking in the morning than adults without ADHD. They also experienced daytime sleepiness more often.

Children with ADHD have also been found to have problems with going to sleep, staying asleep, and waking up in the morning. In addition, they, too, experience excessive daytime sleepiness. ADHD has been generally demonstrated to reduce the time in rapid eye movement (REM) or dream sleep among children while also increasing the frequency of periodic leg movements. There are several theories about the causes of sleep disturbances in people with ADHD. One simple explanation is that the sleep disturbances are directly related to the problems with arousal associated with the ADHD itself.

In addition to insomnia, many adults and children with ADHD report being restless when they sleep, but for some it may be more serious than just tossing and turning. **Restless leg syndrome (RLS)** and sleep-disordered breathing or obstructive sleep apnea are among the more commonly observed sleep disorders in people with ADHD. It seems that people with RLS are more likely to have ADHD than people without RLS. In a 2005 review of clinical studies reporting cases of RLS and ADHD, Cortese and colleagues found that 44% of the adults with ADHD in these studies were found to have RLS, and as many as 26% of individuals with RLS also had ADHD. A similar preliminary study found that 20% of adults with ADHD had RLS compared to 7.2% of those without ADHD. For more on this important topic, you may want to read *100 Questions & Answers About Restless Leg Syndrome* by Sudhansu Chokroverty (Jones & Bartlett Learning, 2011).

Treating ADHD Can Improve Sleep

For years, the association of sleep disorders and ADHD has been overlooked because of the focus on insomnia as a side effect of stimulant medication used to treat ADHD, rather than a coexisting condition. Stimulants may be associated with a delay of sleep onset and insomnia in some people, but in a significant number of patients with ADHD, stimulants may actually improve their ability to fall asleep. In a study by Sobanski and colleagues (2008), 34 adult nonmedicated patients with ADHD were compared to 34 age-matched and sex-matched, medication-free control subjects without psychiatric or sleep disorders. The investigators studied these adults for 2 consecutive nights in the sleep laboratory. When first studied, all 34 adults with ADHD displayed reduced sleep efficiency with longer sleep onset latency and more awakenings. At follow-up, those treated with stimulant medication showed a significant reduction in sleep onset latency and improved sleep efficiency. This study clearly underscores the importance of carefully discussing sleep history with your doctor prior to being treated with stimulants. If it is determined that sleep problems are present prior to the beginning medication and that these problems may possibly be the result of over-arousal, your doctor might prescribe an additional dose of stimulants later in the day or a dosing schedule that provides coverage of symptoms at bedtime.

If problems with sleep persist after adequate treatment of ADHD, however, the clinician may elect to treat problems such as falling asleep with prescription medications. Sleeping pills, however, should be avoided, as the majority of people quickly develop tolerance and they can become habit-forming. Instead, physicians may choose medications with sedative properties that cause sleepiness. These include antihistamines like Benadryl (diphenhydramine) and clonidine or similar drugs administered before bedtime. These medications, however, tend to produce grogginess well into the next day, making getting up the next morning even more difficult. **Melatonin** and **bright light therapy** during the day to regulate sleep/wake cycles have also been tried and proven to be somewhat effective in treating insomnia in both children and adults with ADHD.

Linda speaks:

In addition to my symptoms of ADHD, I have a great deal of difficulty settling down to go to sleep in the evening. As soon as I get in bed, I develop a crawling sensation in my legs and feel like I need to get up and move around. In the morning, my bedclothes are a mess with everything tossed everywhere. The comforter is never on the bed any more. I have always been a restless sleeper, since I was a child, but this is worse.

89. Does lack of sleep or disrupted sleep as a result of various sleep disorders negatively affect ADHD?

Lack of sleep can lead to inattention, behavioral problems, and impaired academic performance in children. Cognitive impairments, diminished executive functioning, and excessive daytime sleepiness have all been reported to be common consequences of **sleep disorders** in adults. Adding these deficits and the physical stress of sleep deprivation to the ADHD symptoms can significantly worsen already-impaired functioning. ADHD and sleep disorders commonly overlap (see the answer to Question 88). Therefore, the need to correctly diagnose and treat both disorders cannot be overemphasized.

Studies have demonstrated that sleep-related breathing disorders were found more frequently in the inattentive/hyperactive children. One study reported that excessive snoring, which may be highly indicative of **obstructive sleep apnea (OSA)**, occurred in 33% of an ADHD population versus 9% in a non-ADHD population. Adults with ADHD may also have problems with snoring and excessive daytime sleepiness; however, they are often unaware that these symptoms may indicate a sleep disorder. Many adults and parents of children with ADHD pass off their snoring and breath pausing as normal and fail to bring it to their doctor's attention. Because the incidence of **sleep apnea** increases with age, sleep problems should be ruled out as the source of daytime sleepiness, inattention, and lack of alertness in adults. To reduce the impact of disordered sleep and lack of sleep on a person with ADHD, physicians should screen for sleep disorders, particularly obstructive sleep apnea, when a patient with ADHD reports excessive daytime sleepiness and fatigue. A sleep study is the preferred method for confirming the diagnosis of sleep disturbances and should be undertaken in all individuals with ADHD with snoring and excessive daytime sleepiness.

A sleep study is the preferred method for confirming the diagnosis of sleep disturbances and should be undertaken in all individuals with ADHD with snoring and excessive daytime sleepiness.

ATHLETICS

90. How does ADHD affect the ability to perform in individual or team athletic endeavors for adults or children with ADHD?

The need for stimulation and increased distractibility can wreak havoc with the plans of any adult or child who wants to set up a regular exercise program or to play a team sport. The tendency to give up if a task is boring can undermine the best of intentions. The solution to this problem often rests in the choice of exercise (or sport) and in personal motivation. Walking on a treadmill is so boring for most women that it will be quickly abandoned without outside stimulation like music or TV to hold their attention. Playing softball and being assigned to the outfield can become a significant problem if a girl with ADHD can not stay focused while waiting for the next fly ball or her turn at bat. However, other sports that offer continuous activity and stimulation like soccer or swimming may not be so problematic. Step aerobics, dancing, ballet, gymnastics, or any activity that builds in socialization with exercise may make it easier for women and girls with ADHD to make a commitment and keep at it.

Despite these inherent difficulties, sports participation has been shown to decrease anxiety and depression in children with ADHD. Athletics can often become an arena for success for children and young adults who have struggled academically and/or socially. Michael Phelps, Olympic gold medalist, is the most shining example of this phenomenon. Swimming became his "island of competence" and allowed him to focus and excel. Practice and meets lent structure to his days and provided him an outlet for his hyperactivity.

Athletics can often become an arena for success for children and young adults who have struggled academically and/or socially.

Studies have shown that aerobic exercise can increase brain neurotrans- mitters, result- ing in an increase in attention and a decrease in hyperactivity.

In addition to the inherent physical and psychological benefits, studies have shown that aerobic exercise can increase brain neurotransmitters, resulting in an increase in attention and a decrease in hyperactivity. John Ratey, MD, in his 2008 book, *Spark: The Revolutionary New Science of Exercise and the Brain*, details how exercise can "build and condition the brain" (p. 3) and that "(W)ith regular exercise, we can raise the baseline levels of dopamine and norepinephrine by spurring the growth of certain receptors in the brain" (p. 158). He even goes so far as to state that for a very small handful of individuals with attention-deficit hyperactivity disorder, exercise may actually be a replacement for stimulants, but for most, it is complementary—something they should absolutely do, along with takings medicines, to help increase attention and improve moods.

SCHOOL

91. What can be done to help parents and teachers recognize what girls with ADHD look like in the classroom?

I have written a great deal in previous answers about the issues of underrecognition and lack of referral of girls with ADHD. (See Questions 8 and 9 for a further discussion.) One of the primary reasons for this situation, however, may have been uncovered by a national survey that measured perceptions about ADHD (Quinn & Wigal, 2004). In this survey, 40% of teachers reported that they were unable to identify girls with ADHD, and only 10% stated that they had received adequate training in recognizing ADHD.

To address this issue, let's turn to ways we can improve the identification of ADHD in girls. In the classroom, girls with ADHD often display the symptoms of

ADHD differently than boys. Teachers and parents, therefore, need to become familiar with these different signs of ADHD in order to identify girls and refer them for evaluation. How does a girl with combined subtype ADHD or inattentive subtype ADHD demonstrate her symptoms in the classroom? The following list may be helpful for teachers (and parents) in identifying girls who may need to be referred for a more comprehensive evaluation.

Symptoms of ADHD combined subtype in girls may be seen in the classroom as:

- Being hypersocial or hypertalkative rather than hyperactive.
- Fidgeting, frequent teacher solicitation, and messiness.
- Blaming others for their mistakes and forgetfulness.
- Rushing through assignments, often with careless errors. These girls may misread directions or start an assignment before the directions are completed.
- Chewing on their fingers, twirling their hair, or tapping a pencil rather than moving around the room.
- Frequently interrupting others in conversation, acting bossy, or failing to pick up on nonverbal cues.
- Easily losing their temper.
- Exhibiting verbal aggression toward peers rather than the physical aggression seen in males. However, they are usually not verbally aggressive toward the teacher and other adults in authority (oppositional defiant disorder), which appears more commonly in males with ADHD.

Despite these behaviors, a girl with ADHD will not be disruptive and will show a general compliance of all classroom rules.

Teachers need to become familiar with these different signs of ADHD in order to identify girls and refer them for evaluations.

Other Issues

Girls with inattentive subtype ADHD may exhibit the following symptoms in the classroom:

- Being messy and disorganized.
- Often making careless mistakes on tests, homework, or in-class work.
- Appearing disheveled.
- Forgetting or losing their personal possessions.
- Often not finishing seat assignments.
- Being off track when called upon by the teacher.
- Asking the teacher or seatmates frequent questions about what they should be doing.
- Having trouble following multistep directions.
- Exhibiting poor test performance when compared to in-class work.
- Frequently forgetting their homework or turning it in late.
- Appearing shy and withdrawn in class.
- Not participating in class discussion.
- Having frequent somatic complaints like headaches or stomachaches, as well as frequent absences.

Girls with ADHD are often required to repeat a grade.

As a result of these problems, particularly lack of readiness, delays in executive functioning, organization and, time management, girls with ADHD are often required to repeat a grade. Seeing their immaturity and skill deficits, the educational system offers grade retention as the solution. Grade retention was seen in 14% of girls with ADHD combined subtype and 20.5% of the inattentive subtype compared with only 3.5% of girls without ADHD in a study of elementary school aged girls with ADHD. This solution, however, is unfortunate. Deficits in executive functioning and organization skills are inherent to ADHD, and the majority of these girls will not develop these critical skills by merely repeating a grade. For most girls with ADHD, such solutions are futile until their ADHD is recognized, properly diagnosed, and treated with a comprehensive, multimodal program including medication, behavioral therapy, appropriate educational placement, and skill development.

Phoebe's mother speaks:

My (immature) daughter is about to turn 12. She does things like fixing herself (hair, etc.) beautifully at home, at night, but during the day, in front of friends, she refuses to even part her hair evenly. She is messy and disorganized and makes careless mistakes. Each year, we have to decide whether to pass her to the next grade, because she's such an underachiever and acts like she doesn't care. I need her to see that she can do better than below average. Her teachers seem at a loss for how to help her.

92. What techniques work best for girls with ADHD in the classroom?

Structure and predictability within the classroom are often the best antidotes to the internal confusion and disorganization that girls with ADHD experience. When it comes to improving their performance, girls with ADHD need well-defined classroom expectations. Organized teachers are, therefore, essential to the success of girls with ADHD and something that parents may want to request when their daughter has ADHD. As one girl stated about such a teacher, "With her, I always know what to expect." In addition, an understanding and supportive classroom teacher can provide the motivation to help these girls perform their best.

Structure and predictability within the classroom are often the best antidotes to the internal confusion and disorganization that girls with ADHD experience.

An understanding and supportive classroom teacher can provide the motivation to help these girls perform their best.

Other Issues

What Motivates Girls with ADHD to Do Well Academically?

Combined subtype ADHD is most often motivated by competition and stimulation, while the inattentive subtype seems to be motivated by teacher approval.

Studies show that combined subtype and inattentive subtype students with ADHD are motivated differently. Combined subtype ADHD is most often motivated by competition and stimulation, while inattentive subtype seems to be motivated by teacher approval. For girls with combined subtype ADHD, teachers can improve classroom behaviors by offering them approved reasons to move around, as well as provide them with leadership roles in the classroom. Keeping in mind that girls with ADHD need to move around, teachers can actively help them identify constructive uses for free time and allow nondistracting fidgeting at their desks. In addition, teachers need to recognize that much of the impulsive behavior seen in these girls is beyond their control and thus should set aside time to problem solve rather than punish them.

The following lists contain other suggestions based on diagnosis for motivating girls with ADHD to do well academically.

Combined Subtype

- Encourage them to compete with themselves, for example: "Let's see if you can complete this assignment or homework with fewer errors, in less time, etc."
- Offer more challenging work that may be more interesting and stimulating.
- Make classwork interactive.
- Set up class teams.
- Give recognition and offer prizes and rewards for work well done.
- Reward effort not just achievement.

Inattentive Subtype

- Provide calm, reassurance to counteract anxiety.
- Emphasize what they *can* do, not what they *can't!*
- Offer frequent verbal cues to refocus attention.
- Praise them for their efforts, not just production or correctness.
- Encourage them—understanding that they can feel easily overwhelmed.
- Teach them to problem solve and develop compensatory strategies.
- Help them avoid embarrassment in the classroom. Develop secret signals to direct their attention rather than calling their names aloud in class, which may embarrass them.

Parents can also help a girl with ADHD be more successful academically by providing emotional support. This includes using encouragement to increase desired behaviors rather than admonishment and criticism. Whenever possible, teachers and parents should demonstrate their caring, concern, and belief in the girl with ADHD. This requires both paying attention to and magnifying the small stuff. Parents (and teachers) can also encourage the girl with ADHD to participate in finding solutions to her problems. This creates buy-in while making her feel that her voice and opinion matter. When problems do develop in the classroom, however, a teacher can calmly remove the girl from the situation and discuss options and possible solutions. By helping her understand that we all make mistakes and what to do when we make them, the adults in her life can help a girl with ADHD build problem-solving skills as well as maintain her self-esteem. To avoid such situations altogether, it may also be important to anticipate the trigger points for problems or keep in mind transitional difficulties.

In addition, when addressing academic success, teachers and parents should remember to emphasize learning over performance. To improve achievement, a girl might be allowed to do extra credit work to counterbalance a low test score or to retake tests to demonstrate that she has learned the material. Teachers should understand that efficiency and productivity are affected by ADHD and allow extra time on tests or for the completion of assignments. Last, adults should all encourage girls with ADHD to focus on areas of interest and ability where they are more likely to do better.

93. Why does it seem that some girls do well until college and then have things fall apart?

Girls with ADHD are often able to compensate for their ADHD symptoms for many years.

As noted previously (see Question 10), girls with ADHD are often able to compensate for their ADHD symptoms for many years. They spend a great deal of time and effort and seek help from others in order to function and cope with academic and social demands. In addition, many girls (and women) develop perfectionist qualities or obsessive-compulsive–like behaviors in order to keep their ADHD symptoms under control. They make lists or develop habits or rituals to compensate for their deficits (see Question 58 for a more in-depth discussion of these obsessive-compulsive or perfectionistic behaviors and why they occur). These strategies tend to serve them well and allow for successful academic performance as long as they are living at home and have someone to assist with other tasks such as laundry, food preparation, shopping, and so forth, giving them more time to devote to studying. Friendships and social life are easier and require less effort in high school as these girls usually associate and form friendships with girls from school or an after-school activity.

Adjustment to college, however, is difficult for students with ADHD, and studies have documented that they have more academic concerns and depression than students without ADHD. When young women with ADHD arrive at college, they are on their own and must do everything for themselves! This includes making decisions about which groups to join, who to become friends with, and all the other activities of daily living including when to get up and when to go to bed. They need to get to the cafeteria or shop for and cook their own food as well as handle money and keep track of finances, sometimes for the first time. These extra daily chores and activities, in addition to the increased academic demands of college, place a great deal of stress on their time-management and decision-making skills. Often, at this point, the burden becomes too great and these young women crumble under the load—either becoming severely depressed or simply overwhelmed and paralyzed—unable to function at all. If they are fortunate, a late diagnosis of ADHD is made, and steps can be taken to put a plan in place for a successful recovery. However, for others it is not uncommon that they are misdiagnosed with depression, or not diagnosed at all, and drop out or are invited to leave college.

If they are fortunate, a primary care physician or family pediatrician can look beyond their charm and past academic success and accurately diagnose the ADHD that lies underneath these problems, but for many, this never happens, and they wander along never quite living up to their potential.

These extra daily chores and activities, in addition to the increased academic demands of college, place a great deal of stress on their time-management and decision-making skills.

Other Issues

Isabelle, Tatiana's mother, speaks:

After 15 years of struggling in school, my 20-year-old daughter was recently diagnosed with inattentive type ADHD. She simply could not adapt to the unstructured environment at college, making it impossible for her to succeed. After many tests, the psychiatrist diagnosed her and prescribed Concerta [methylphenidate]. However, my daughter continues to have feelings of boredom, low self-esteem, and laziness when her medication wears off at the end of the day. This is causing her to reject the medication, but most of these symptoms were present in her even before she started taking medication. She needs more help. Can she get it at college?

Emily speaks:

I have really bad ADD and have had since about 5th grade. I am currently a senior in high school and moving on to college in the fall. I have switched from medication to medication and none of it seems to be working in the way that would greatly help me. I also suffer from depression and I'm on medication for that, too. How can I relax and not worry so much about schoolwork and stop being afraid that I won't graduate or flunk out in college because I lack the ability to stay on task? I need a plan!

94. How can someone with ADHD be sure she is choosing the right college?

The answer to this question very much hinges on two things—first, the maturity and level of independence of the young woman with ADHD, and second, the accessibility and amount of support available at the institution. While each student is different, good grades in high school may not be the best predictor of success in college. Often, those grades were earned with a lot of support from various adults in the young woman's

Good grades in high school may not be the best predictor of success in college.

life, by the structure provided in high school, and the differing academic expectations in high school versus college. As pointed out in the answer to the previous question, a lack of maturity may become all too clear as young women with ADHD try to navigate on their own in college.

How to Choose a College and Ensure Success

In addition to skills, it is important for you and your family to assess if you are a good match for the college or university you are considering and whether the institution has the appropriate level of services for you. Having a plan and gathering as much information as possible about the institution will allow you to answer both questions. First, make a list of the top four or five colleges you are considering attending. Next, visit the admissions Web sites of each institution. Most Web sites will list the course requirements that entering seniors must have completed to apply to the college. This list will help you look at the courses you should be taking in high school. There are also several popular published catalogs that you can buy or borrow from the library that may have this type of information on colleges. Next, make a table of all the facts you have gathered. At this point you should have a good idea of your chances for being accepted to one of these colleges.

After you have evaluated the prospects for acceptance, it is time to visit the colleges in person. It is never too early to get on a college campus and get a firsthand look at what this new world will be like. At all of the campuses you visit, it is critical that you schedule a visit to the office on each campus that deals with students with ADHD as well as any other support services offices. Many colleges offer more than services, and accommodations for students with diagnosed disabilities.

It is never too early to get on a college campus and get a firsthand look at what this new world will be like.

Some also have tutoring programs, writing and/or learning centers, and counseling programs. This is the time to get a firsthand look at these resources. If at all possible, ask the person in charge of serving students with ADHD if any students with these disabilities would be available to talk with you. A face-to-face discussion with a college student who has similar disabilities can be very enlightening.

A face-to-face discussion with a college student who has similar disabilities can be very enlightening.

Last, you need to be knowledgeable about your own strengths and weaknesses and your ADHD. You cannot be too prepared regarding these issues prior to attending college. The transition to college can be extremely difficult, and the more practice and information you have ahead of time, the better the outcome will be. You will need to be responsible for your medication, doctor visits, and prescriptions. In addition, you will need to advocate for yourself with professors and the students with disabilities office. At college, you must self-disclose and seek services on your own. No one will be looking out for you on campus or seeing if you are attending class or accessing accommodations. You must see the value of your treatment plan and continue to pursue the path that leads to success on your own.

Frank, Jennifer's father, speaks:

My daughter went to the local state university for a year and a half. She did okay at first, but she started slipping after freshman midterms. But she ended up okay. Second semester freshman year she failed about half her courses. My wife and I suspected ADD, so we took her to a specialist, and she was immediately diagnosed and put on medication. After diagnosis, we were able to get her bad grades withdrawn and her scholarships restored. We got her hooked up with the school's DSS (disabled student services) office and thought that that would be the end of it! It turns out that the school's policy is that the student must be proactive in making and keeping appointments with the DSS counselor. Being new to ADD, we did not know how this would work against her. Had we known we would have insisted that out daughter sign the waiver which allowed the counselor to keep parents in the loop regarding her compliance to the program that had been put into place for her. What we found out after the semester ended was that my daughter stopped going to classes about halfway through her third semester, shortly after she stopped taking her medication and stopped seeing the counselor. She failed everything! The lesson we learned is that there needs to be some accountability and that my daughter needed more help. She was definitely not ready to do it on her own. Just having the diagnosis of ADD was not enough!

PART FIVE

Getting More Help for ADHD

Should a woman with ADHD hire a professional
organizer to help with household tasks?

How do I choose a coach?

What is an ADHD-friendly lifestyle?

More . . .

95. Should a woman with ADHD hire a professional organizer to help her sort through her clutter and get better organized at home?

When a woman with ADHD is trying to get more organized, a professional organizer can definitely make all the difference.

Women who have ADHD are often in need of this type of organizational support as they often do not have the skills necessary to organize their environment.

When a woman with ADHD is trying to get more organized, **a professional organizer** can definitely make all the difference. A professional organizer, who specializes in working with adults with ADHD, can be a virtual lifesaver. They can teach you the basic organizational skills necessary to get your home organized and to keep it that way. Women who have ADHD are often in need of this type of organizational support as they often do not have the skills necessary to organize their environment. However, finding the professional organizer, who both understands ADHD and meets your specific needs, may not be as easy as it sounds.

Different organizers, depending on their training, may have different approaches to the organizing process. Some organizers work strictly through coaching, helping you to set goals and to find systems that work best for you (and ways to stick to them). Others may have a more hands-on approach, helping you organize on-site; and sometimes they use a combination of both strategies. When considering hiring a professional organizer, you should discuss these various methods as well as the organizer's background and training. Inquire about their experiences working with clients with ADHD in the past, what worked and what did not, and what they know about ADHD. Asking how they think ADHD affects organizational skills and what methods, in their opinion, work best when someone has ADHD will give you some insight as to whether you think this is the right person for you. Be a wise consumer and ask for references and contact information for previous clients. Discuss fees and be sure you come to a clear understanding of what will be involved in the process of organizing your home. Set specific goals and be clear about what you are looking to accomplish before beginning the relationship with any organizer. More information on professional organizing can be found on the Web site of the National Association of Professional Organizers at www.napo.net.

96. What is coaching and how does it help when a person has ADHD?

The concept of **coaching** has been around for a long time. Coaching takes place in many arenas, but is probably best known in athletics. Coaching can be provided by tutors, mentors, or any other person in a supportive role. Recently, however, coaching has taken on a new meaning, particularly in the world of business. Life skills or professional coaching has proven quite effective in helping to achieve or manage a successful career. The concept of coaching was first introduced to the ADHD community in the book, *Driven to Distraction: Recognizing and Coping With Attention-Deficit Disorder From Childhood Through Adulthood*, written in 1995 by Drs. Edward Hallowell and John Ratey.

An **ADHD coach** is a person knowledgeable about ADHD and skilled in the process of helping you maximize your strengths and talents and take action toward reaching your goals. He or she can help you set realistic short- and long-term goals, problem solve, and stay on track as you work to make changes and achieve these goals. By using a process of inquiry, the ADHD coach can help you identify problems, brainstorm appropriate solutions, and put those solutions into action. ADHD coaching is a partnership that

He or she can help you set realistic short- and long-term goals, problem solve, and stay on track as you work to make changes and achieve these goals.

ADHD coaching is a partnership that supports you in examining your strengths and weaknesses.

supports you in examining your strengths and weaknesses and helps you to develop the needed strategies to improve your day-to-day functioning. Your ADHD coach can assist you in the process of designing an ADHD-friendly environment that meets your unique needs and thus allows you to "operate in your GREEN zone" and become more productive. (See the answer to Question 99 for a more in-depth explanation of this concept.) In addition to being nonjudgmental and supportive, a coach may also offer suggestions and reminders, establish structure and boundaries, and provide the much-needed aspect of accountability that your life has been lacking. By helping you examine lifestyle issues, a coach can help you make desired changes in areas such as diet, sleep habits, and exercise programs that will foster the optimum health and balance you are seeking. In addition, you will begin working on particular skills and set short-term goals to address areas such as time management and organization, with the coach agreeing to hold you accountable for your actions, thus ensuring that you make steady progress toward those goals.

97. How do I choose a coach?

Once you make the decision to add coaching to your ADHD treatment program, it is important that you take a few additional steps in order to ensure the best possible coach–client match for a successful relationship. Before contacting a coach, reflect on your needs and what you want from the coaching relationship. Many coaches specialize in different areas—time management, organization, workplace issues—or specific clients, for example, college students, adults, or children. In addition, you will need to decide whether it is important for you to meet face-to-face with a coach or whether phone sessions will work for you. Next, gather

Before contacting a coach, reflect on your needs and what you want from the coaching relationship.

the names and contact information for a few coaches from trusted sources (therapists, organization Web sites, or other adults with ADHD). If the coach has a Web site (most do), visit the site and try to assess whether the coach would be a good match for you.

Once you have identified potential coaches, you are ready to set up a phone interview before scheduling an initial meeting. The following questions can be asked during the phone interview to gather more information on the coach before you make a final decision:

- How long have you been involved in ADHD coaching?
- How many clients do you have who have ADHD?
- How do you prefer to work (only face-to-face, by telephone and e-mail, etc.)?
- I have identified _____ as one of my needs. What is your experience in this area?
- How often do you anticipate we would need to meet?
- What are your fees?
- Can you provide me with references (colleagues, former clients, etc.)?
- When would you be available for an initial interview?

After the phone interview you should have a sense of the coach as a person and whether or not you will be able to work with him or her. Check out references and the coach's Web site for more information. Then set up a face-to-face meeting. At this meeting, you can get a sense of how well you would work together and formalize financial arrangements as well as how the coaching sessions will take place (i.e., face-to-face, by e-mail, or by phone). Coaching is a valuable (and expensive) resource. Taking the time to get things right from the beginning will help to ensure that the experience will be a positive one for all involved.

98. How can a woman or girl with ADHD reframe her ADHD?

Women and girls with ADHD are often their own harshest critics.

Women and girls with ADHD are often their own harshest critics. Early on, their life experiences confirm their failure to live up to expectations set by themselves or others. As mentioned previously, they blame themselves for their deficits and feel helpless to make changes in the face of these difficulties. Attempts to conform and their desire to succeed cause them to expend ever greater amounts of time and effort resulting in a sense of being "overwhelmed" and an inability to accomplish what others seem to do effortlessly. Life becomes a vicious cycle where they are less likely to make an effort to attempt or finish tasks, further reinforcing their sense of failure and inability to accomplish goals they have set in life. Even if they do manage, through a great deal of effort, to compensate for their shortcomings, they often feel like imposters or that their competence will be called into question. Challenging this ingrained way of thinking (**reframing**) is essential to changing their self-perception.

Initially, the diagnosis of ADHD itself can provide a great sense of relief for these women and girls by putting a label on what they are experiencing. By viewing their problems and failures through the lens of a real neurobiological disorder and seeing these issues in the larger context of strengths and weaknesses instead of blaming themselves, they often gain a sense of relief. Instead of perceiving their problems as unchangeable, they finally can accept who they are and exchange hope for hopelessness and compassion for criticism.

As part of this process, a woman or girl with ADHD needs to change her perspective and learn to reconsider her behavior in a more positive light. By seeking alternative, ADHD-friendly pathways and feeling comfortable with herself, she will be better able to view life's events as more under her control. By making choices that are best for her, she can reframe her self-expectations and begin to value her uniqueness.

99. What is an ADHD-friendly lifestyle?

An **ADHD-friendly lifestyle** is one in which you draw on your strengths and let them carry you through your weaknesses. As Dr. Kathleen Nadeau often states, "An ADHD-friendly lifestyle is one where you operate in your 'Green zone' as opposed to your 'Red zone.'" Living an ADHD-friendly lifestyle allows you to forgive past mistakes and use humor to get through your present trials as you work with your ADHD instead of always fighting against it. Within this nurturing environment, you are also free to practice extreme self-care and to ask for help when you need it without feeling weak or defective. It is hard enough to be a woman with ADHD without being surrounded by family and friends who blame you for your difficulties! This lifestyle will carry you along whether you are at home with your family and friends or in the workplace.

An ADHD-friendly family is one in which all family members understand the impact of ADHD and work together to find solutions. While family members need to be educated about ADHD and learn to support each other, the household you live in needs to be made ADHD-friendly. ADHD-friendly means low-maintenance, convenient, and less stressful. An ADHD-friendly household has furnishings and floor coverings that are easy to maintain; it has easy, convenient places

A woman or girl with ADHD needs to change her perspective and learn to reconsider her behavior in a more positive light.

An ADHD-friendly lifestyle is one in which you draw on your strengths and let them carry you through your weaknesses.

Living an ADHD-friendly lifestyle allows you to forgive past mistakes.

ADHD-friendly means low-maintenance, convenient, and less stressful.

Getting More Help for ADHD

to hang keys, sort mail, store coats, toys, backpacks, briefcases and so forth, so that they are not just tossed anywhere and misplaced. An ADHD-friendly family recognizes that mom cannot do it all. Chores are assigned to all family members on the basis of preference and ability. ADHD-friendly households are simplified. An ADHD-friendly family is constantly on the watch for stresses that can be reduced or eliminated.

An ADHD-friendly family recognizes that mom cannot do it all.

A second step toward an ADHD-friendly life consists of taking an inventory of friends and associates in your life. As a woman with ADHD, you need to consciously seek out people who appreciate your best qualities and are supportive of you. To make life more ADHD-friendly, you may need to make an unbiased assessment of the people in your life whose messages are negative and destructive and either educate them about ADHD or reduce your contact with them. Being around people who appreciate you will allow you to think of yourself more positively and open the way to happiness and success.

100. Where can I go for more information on ADHD in women and girls?

Information about the National Center for Girls and Women with AD/HD can be found at www. ncgiadd.org.

In 1997, Dr. Kathleen Nadeau and I founded The National Center for Girls and Women with AD/HD (www.ncgiadd.org) to raise awareness, foster research, and advocate for women and girls with ADHD. Our work has met with success, as more girls and women are diagnosed and included in research studies, but much more still needs to be done. If you still have unanswered questions or are seeking more information about ADHD in general, or in women and girls in particular, visit our Web sites: www.ncgiadd.org and www.addvance. com. In addition, there are many other Web sites and free newsletters that we have included in Appendix B of this book.

Taking a Closer Look at DSM-IV-TR and DSM-5

DSM-IV criteria require that a person demonstrates at least six of nine symptoms of inattention, or at least six of nine symptoms of hyperactivity/impulsivity; that these symptoms must have been present for at least 6 months; and that some symptoms were present before the age of 7. In addition, the person must demonstrate some impairment from the symptoms in two or more settings (e.g., at school or work and at home), and there must be **clinically significant impairment** in social, academic, or occupational functioning. The final requirement for diagnosis states that symptoms may not be caused by another or coexisting condition.

Using these DSM-IV-TR criteria, a person may be diagnosed with one of three subtypes of ADHD. These subtypes include:

1. *Predominantly inattentive subtype*—In this subtype, the individual will have six or more symptoms of inattentiveness and/or fewer than six of the symptoms of hyperactivity/impulsivity. Individuals in this subtype will most likely have inattentiveness as a significant clinical feature.

2. *Predominantly hyperactive/impulsive subtype*—In this subtype, the individual will demonstrate six or more symptoms of hyperactivity/impulsivity and fewer than six symptoms of inattentiveness.

3. *Combined subtype*—In this subtype, the individual will demonstrate six or more (out of nine) symptoms in both the inattentive and hyperactive/impulsive categories. This is the most common subtype of ADHD in both children and adults.

The American Psychiatric Association (APA), recognizing the diagnostic problems inherent in DSM-IV-TR, has suggested several proposed changes in DSM-5 (APA, 2010), due out in 2013. These proposed changes include maintaining the present criteria but without subtypes, or discontinuing predominantly hyperactive/impulsive and predominantly inattentive subtypes. It is also entertaining the possibility of making changes to the current inattentive subtype by either creating a new diagnosis of attention-deficit disorder (ADD), with the same inattention criteria that are present in DSM-IV-TR's predominantly inattentive subtype requiring that no hyperactive/impulsivity criteria are present or retaining the current predominantly inattentive subtype but requiring that no more than two hyperactivity criteria contribute to the diagnosis.

The following exercise takes a look at each of the criteria of DSM-IV-TR and provides a more in-depth discussion of the diagnostic picture in females, a critique of each diagnostic criterion of DSM-IV-TR, and the reasons why each misses the mark or fails completely in identifying females. It was first presented in *Gender Issues and AD/HD: Research, Diagnosis and Treatment* (2002), a book I coedited and published with Kathleen Nadeau, PhD, and is expanded and updated here along with the latest DSM-5 proposed changes (APA, 2010).

Symptoms (Criterion A)

This current diagnostic criterion requires that a person exhibit six out of nine symptoms of inattention and/or six out of nine symptoms of hyperactivity-impulsivity and is applied equally to males and females. There are significant problems, however, with expecting that females meet the six-out-of-nine-symptoms criterion needed for a diagnosis in DSM-IV-TR (especially in the hyperactive/impulsive category). The current cutoff for number of symptoms needed for diagnosing ADHD was derived from **field trial research**. The field trials for ADHD were conducted with an inadequate number of girls (80). Such a small sample does not permit a careful study of possible cutoff differences by gender and age group. Another important point is that the children in the field trials for ADHD were clinic-referred and, as has been established in numerous studies, clinic-referred girls with ADHD tend to present with more severe symptoms relative to nonclinic-referred girls with ADHD. Thus, it is unlikely that the sample of girls included in the DSM-IV field trials was representative of the majority of girls with ADHD.

While six or more symptoms in either or both subtypes are required to diagnose ADHD, several studies have shown that older women and girls may have as few as four or five symptoms and have their lives significantly affected. In one particular study conducted at the Children's Hospital of Philadelphia, researchers evaluated 375 girls ages 6 to 13 years referred for a diagnosis of ADHD and looked at both functional impairment and coexisting conditions. In order to assess functional impairment at the **subthreshold level** (four to five symptoms), girls were divided according to the symptoms of ADHD endorsed on a standardized **rating scale** completed by their parents and compared to girls in a group that met DSM-IV-TR criterion (≥6 symptoms) and a control group without ADHD. Results indicated that girls in the inattentive or combined subthreshold groups demonstrated significant functional impairment as rated by parents and clinicians. Sixty-one percent of girls in the inattentive subthreshold group, and 67% of girls in the combined subthreshold group demonstrated impairment in at least two domains and did not differ from girls in the DSM group with regard to social skills, adaptability, study skills, and homework problems completed. Girls in the combined subthreshold group did not differ from girls in the DSM group with regard to social skills, adaptability, study skills, and global impairment. Girls in the inattentive subthreshold group did not differ from their counterparts in the DSM groups in coexisting mood and anxiety disorders. Girls in the DSM combined group had significantly higher rates of externalizing disorders; however, 22% of girls in the combined subthreshold group did meet criteria for a disruptive disorder. Overall, it seems that results from this study indicate that girls with scores in the subthreshold range (four to five symptoms) do demonstrate significant functional impairments and are similar to girls with a DSM diagnosis ($\geq$6 symptoms) and should, therefore, also be diagnosed with ADHD.

The manifestations of adult ADHD are likewise not well represented by the criteria. The symptoms as currently endorsed describe the disorder as it presents in elementary school-aged children, and these descriptions are often not relevant to what is going on in the lives of adults. The APA in its proposed changes to DSM-5 for the Diagnostic Criteria for Attention Deficit/Hyperactivity Disorder (http://www.dsm5.org/ProposedRevisions/Pages/proposedrevision.aspx?rid=383) has recognized this limitation and has proposed an elaboration of each existing symptom that makes each more relevant for adults. For example, the symptom, "Is often on the go or often acts as if driven by a motor" would have the following elaboration for adults: "is averse to being still for extended time, feels [he or she] has to get going when in restaurants, during lectures; is perceived as being hard to keep up with, as being too restless; has difficulty unwinding or relaxing" (http://www.dsm5.org/Proposed Revisions/Pages/proposedrevision.aspx?rid=383). In addition, it has been well-documented that many of the symptoms of ADHD decrease over time while impairment remains. Adults with ADHD have been shown to demonstrate significant impairment with fewer symptoms. Taking this fact into consideration, APA has proposed that in DSM-5, the symptom threshold may be lowered from 6 to 3 endorsed criteria from each subtype for adults. It also proposes to add more impulsive symptoms, making them equal to inattentive and hyperactive symptoms.

In addition, rating scales used to help identify the disorder often rely on cutoff scores to determine the severity of symptoms such as hyperactivity. This presents a problem for the diagnosis in females because girls with ADHD have been found to exhibit lower symptom severity for inattention, hyperactivity, and impulsivity than boys in studies of both general population and clinic-referred samples. As a result, girls with ADHD would have to exhibit greater symptom severity than boys in order to be diagnosed with ADHD. Girls without hyperactive symptoms are more difficult to diagnose and can be easily overlooked. Furthermore, it appears that symptoms of inattentiveness are more stable across the life span than hyperactive symptoms, which appear to be more characteristic of younger children. Thus, adolescent girls and women with ADHD are less likely to display these symptoms. In addition, many of the symptoms listed in DSM-IV-TR are seen as more male-oriented. In a study that had mothers rate the symptoms of ADHD as masculine or feminine, "talks excessively" was the only symptom they considered to be a feminine trait.

Age of Onset (Criterion B)

Some hyperactive-impulsive or inattentive symptoms that caused impairment were present before the age of 7 years. The later onset of symptoms seen in girls with ADHD makes it important to address this criterion. Earlier onset of symptoms is usually associated with hyperactivity, more severe symptoms, and poorer school performance. Protective factors and lack of disruptive behaviors may delay the diagnosis in girls. DSM-5 has proposed to change this criterion and raise the age of onset to 12 years.

Functional Impairment (Criterion C)

Some impairment from symptoms is present in two or more settings (e.g., at school or work and at home). Girls and women often work harder to compensate for and or hide their ADHD symptoms. Therefore, impairment for them may often be one of degree or the amount of time and effort it takes for a girl or woman with ADHD to maintain normalcy. In addition, a girl or woman's impairment in functioning may be more readily determined by comparing her overall functioning to others in her peer group or at home rather than looking at her academic achievement. Evidence of ADHD is often less likely to be found on the report cards of girls with ADHD for a variety of reasons. Girls tend to work harder to meet teacher expectations. Inattention often goes unrecognized if a girl learns to look at the teacher and has no disruptive behavior. Thus, satisfactory performance and academic achievement in school cannot rule out ADHD in females.

Clinically Significant Impairment (Criterion D)

There must be clear evidence of clinically significant impairment in social, academic, or occupational functioning. This criterion requiring that ADHD be clinically significant often confuses the diagnosis with a disability determination. In previous versions of the DSM and for other diagnoses there is no requirement for degree of impairment or that the individual present with impaired functioning in multiple settings. For a great many disorders, varying degrees of impairment along a continuum from mild to severe are recognized, and distinctions are acknowledged between the requirements for diagnosis versus disability. For example, no one would argue with a diagnosis of mild or moderate depression and require that the affected individual be significantly disabled and unable to work or perform in school.

Coexisting Conditions (Criterion E)

The symptoms . . . are not better accounted for by another mental disorder. It has been well established that ADHD rarely occurs alone. Seventy-five percent of adults with ADHD have at least one other psychiatric condition, usually depression. While this criterion is meant to prevent the misdiagnosis of ADHD, in adults with ADHD the opposite is often true; coexisting conditions are diagnosed while the ADHD goes undiagnosed. Women with ADHD are commonly diagnosed correctly or incorrectly with depression, and the ADHD, the sole or coexisting diagnosis, is missed. While the presence of coexisting disorders in individuals with ADHD is more likely than not, it is important that clinicians familiarize themselves with the symptoms of ADHD that mimic these conditions in order to avoid missing the diagnosis of ADHD itself.

Taking a Closer Look at DSM-IV-TR and DSM-5

Resources

Books Written Specifically for Girls and Women with ADHD

The Adventures of Phoebe Flowers: Stories of a Girl With AD/HD
Barbara Roberts
Washington, DC: Advantage Books, 2010

Attention, Girls! A Guide to Learn About Your ADHD
Patricia O. Quinn, MD
Washington, DC: Magination Press, 2009

Gender Issues and AD/HD: Research, Diagnosis and Treatment
Patricia O. Quinn, MD, and Kathleen Nadeau, PhD (Editors)
Washington, DC: Advantage Books, 2002

The Girls' Guide to AD/HD
Beth Walker
Bethesda, MD: Woodbine House, 2005

Moms With ADD: A Self-Help Manual
Christine A. Adamec
Lanham, MD: Taylor Trade Publishing, 2000

Survival Tips for Women With AD/HD: Beyond Piles, Palms & Post-its
Terry Matlen, MSW
Plantation, FL: Specialty Press, Inc., 2005

Understanding Girls With AD/HD
Kathleen, G. Nadeau, PhD, Ellen Littman, PhD, and Patricia O. Quinn, MD
Washington, DC: Advantage Books, 1999

Understanding Women With AD/HD
Kathleen G. Nadeau, PhD, and Patricia O. Quinn, MD (Editors)
Washington, DC: Advantage Books, 2002

When Moms and Kids Have ADD (expanded version)
Patricia O. Quinn, MD, and Kathleen G. Nadeau, PhD
Washington, DC: Advantage Books, 2004

*Women With Attention Deficit Disorder: Embrace Your Differences and Transform
Your Life*
Sari Solden, MS, LMFT
Nevada City, CA: Underwood Books, 1995, 2005

Books to Help Women Understand and Cope with Their ADHD

*A Housekeeper Is Cheaper Than a Divorce: Why You CAN Afford to Hire Help and
How to Get It*
Kathy Fitzgerald Sherman
Mountain View, CA: Life Tools Press, 2000

ADD and Romance: Finding Fulfillment in Love, Sex & Relationships
Jonathan Scott Halverstadt, MS
Lanham, MD: Taylor Trade Publishing, 1998

ADD in the Workplace: Choices, Changes and Challenges
Kathleen G. Nadeau, PhD
New York, NY: Taylor & Francis Group, 1997

AD/HD-Friendly Ways to Organize Your Life
Judith Kolberg and Kathleen Nadeau, PhD
New York, NY: Taylor & Francis Group, 2002

*The Disorganized Mind: Coaching Your ADHD Brain to Take Control of Your
Time, Tasks, and Talents*
Nancy Ratey, EdM, MCC, SCAC
New York, NY: St. Martin's Press, 2008

Driven to Distraction: Recognizing and Coping With Attention Deficit Disorder From Childhood Through Adulthood
Edward M. Hallowell, MD, and John J. Ratey, MD
New York, NY: Touchstone Publishing, 1995

Finding a Career That Works for You: A Step-by-Step Guide to Choosing a Career
Wilma R. Fellman, MEd, LPC
Plantation, FL: Specialty Press, Inc., 2006

Is It You, Me, or Adult A.D.D.? Stopping the Roller Coaster When Someone You Love Has Attention Deficit Disorder
Gina Pera
San Francisco, CA: 1201 Alarm Press, 2008

More Attention, Less Deficit: Success Strategies for Adults With ADHD
Ari Tuckman, PsyD
Plantation, FL: Specialty Press, Inc., 2009

Odd One Out: The Maverick's Guide to Adult ADD
Jennifer Koretsky
Plattekill, NY: Vervante, 2007

Organizing Solutions for People With Attention Deficit Disorder: Tips and Tools to Help You Take Charge of Your Life and Get Organized
Susan C. Pinsky
Beverly, MA: Fair Winds Press, 2006

Pieces of a Puzzle: The Link Between Eating Disorders and ADD
Carolyn Piver Dukarm, MD
Washington, DC: Advantage Books, 2006

What Does Everybody Else Know That I Don't? Social Skills Help for Adults With Attention Deficit/Hyperactivity Disorder
Michelle Novonti, PhD
Plantation, FL: Specialty Press, Inc., 1999

Books to Help You Parent Your Child or Teen with ADHD

1-2-3 Magic: Effective Discipline for Children 2–12
Thomas W. Phelan, PhD
Glen Ellyn, IL: ParentMagic, Inc., 2004

From Chaos to Calm: Effective Parenting for Challenging Children With ADHD and Other Behavior Problems
Janet E. Heininger, PhD, and Sharon K. Weiss, MEd
New York, NY: Perigee Trade, 2001

Our Family Meeting Book: Fun and Easy Ways to Manage Time, Build Communication, and Share Responsibility Week by Week
Elaine Hightower and Betsy Riley
Minneapolis, MN: Free Spirit Publishing, 2002

Raise Your Child's Social IQ: Stepping Stones to People Skills for Kids
Cathi Cohen, LCSW
Washington, DC: Advantage Books, 2000

Ready for Take-Off: Preparing Your Teen With AD/HD or LD for College
Theresa Maitland, PhD, and Patricia O. Quinn, MD
Washington, DC: Magination Press, 2010

Surviving Your Adolescents
Thomas W. Phelan, PhD
Glen Ellyn, IL: ParentMagic, Inc., 1998

Understanding Girls With AD/HD
Kathleen, G. Nadeau, PhD, Ellen Littman, PhD, and Patricia O. Quinn, MD
Washington, DC: Advantage Books, 1999

Books to Help Your Child Understand and Live with Her ADHD

50 Activities and Games for Kids With ADHD
Patricia O. Quinn, MD, and Judith M. Stern, MA
Washington, DC: Magination Press, 2000

Annie's Plan: Taking Charge of Schoolwork and Homework
Jeanne Kraus
Washington, DC: Magination Press, 2007

Attention, Girls! A Guide to Learn About Your ADHD
Patricia O. Quinn, MD
Washington, DC: Magination Press, 2009

Learning to Slow Down and Pay Attention (Third edition)
Kathleen G. Nadeau, PhD, and Ellen B. Dixon, PhD
Washington, DC: Magination Press, 2005

The "Putting on the Brakes" Activity Book for Kids With ADD or ADHD
   (Second edition)
Patricia O. Quinn, MD, and Judith M. Stern, MA
Washington, DC: Magination Press, 2009

Putting on the Brakes: Understanding and Taking Control of Your ADD or ADHD
   (Second edition)
Patricia O. Quinn, MD, and Judith M. Stern, MA
Washington, DC: Magination Press, 2009

The Survival Guide for Kids With ADD or ADHD
John F. Taylor, PhD
Minneapolis, MN: Free Spirit Publishing, 2006

Books to Help Your Teenager or College Student Cope with Her ADHD

*ADD and the College Student: A Guide for High School and College Students With
   Attention Deficit Disorder* (Revised edition)
Patricia O. Quinn, MD (Editor)
Washington, DC: Magination Press, 2001

The Girls' Guide to AD/HD
Beth Walker
Bethesda, MD: Woodbine House, 2005

Help4ADD@High School (Second edition)
Kathleen G. Nadeau, PhD
Washington, DC: Advantage Books, 2010

Ready for Take-Off: Preparing Your Teen With AD/HD or LD for College
Theresa Maitland, PhD and Patricia O. Quinn, MD
Washington, DC: Magination Press, 2010

Survival Guide for College Students With ADHD or LD (Second edition)
Kathleen G. Nadeau, PhD
Washington, DC: Magination Press, 2006

Resources

Organizations That Provide Help to Women and Families With ADHD

ADD Research Update

This site helps you get updated on the latest ADD (ADHD) research and
information.
www.helpforadd.com

ADHD Aware

ADHD Aware was founded with the conviction that the needs of the ADHD
community are unique, substantial, and worthy of attention. As a nonprofit
organization, its purpose is to strengthen families, cultivate leadership, and
philanthropy, and to foster respect for all individuals by providing services that
contribute to the health and vitality of the community as a whole.
P.O. Box 459
Doylestown, PA 18901
E-mail: info@adhdaware.org
ADHDaware.org

Attention-Deficit Disorder (ADD) Resources

ADD Resources is a nonprofit membership organization to help people with
ADHD achieve their full potential through education and support.
223 Tacoma Avenue South, No. 100
Tacoma, WA 98402
Telephone: (253) 759-5085
Fax: (253) 572-3700
www.addresources.org

Children and Adults with Attention-Deficit/Hyperactivity Disorder (CHADD)

A national advocacy organization for children and adults with ADD, CHADD
has a highly informative Web site with scientifically accurate information as
well as an online bookstore. CHADD also maintains a federally funded ADD
resource center staffed by individuals available to answer your questions and to
help you find the resources that you need.
8181 Professional Place, Suite 201
Landover, MD 20785
Telephone: (800) 233-4050
Fax: (301) 306-7090
www.chadd.org

Edge Foundation

The foundation's mission is to help every child, adolescent, and young adult with attention-deficit hyperactivity disorder to fully realize his or her own potential, personal vision, and passion. The staff at the Edge Foundation believes that professional coaching, while not a substitute for the traditional multimodal treatment for ADHD, is a critical and highly effective intervention in the nontraditional learner's ability to realize his or her potential.

2017 Fairview Avenue East, Suite I
Seattle WA 98102
Telephone: (888) 718-8886
Fax: (877) 718-2220
E-mail: info@edgefoundation.org
www.edgefoundation.org

Kathleen G. Nadeau, PhD

Chesapeake ADHD Center of Maryland
8607 Cedar Street
Silver Spring, MD 20910
Telephone: (301) 562-8448
Fax: (301) 562-8449
www.chesapeakeadd.com

National Attention Deficit Disorder Association (ADDA)

A nonprofit advocacy organization that focuses on issues of teens, adults, and families with ADD. Membership includes a bimonthly newsletter, *Focus*, and discounts at the annual national meeting.

P.O. Box 543
Pottstown, PA 19464
Telephone: (484) 945-2101
Fax: (610) 970-7520
www.add.org

National Center for Girls and Women with AD/HD

An organization that advocates for women and girls with AD/HD. The site includes articles specifically focused on the unique issues faced by women and girls.

3268 Arcadia Place, NW
Washington, DC 20015
Telephone: (888) 238-8588
Fax: (202) 966-1561
www.ncgiadd.org

The National Resource Center on AD/HD

This program of CHADD has been established with funding from the U.S. Centers for Disease Control and Prevention (CDC) to be a national clearinghouse of information and resources concerning this important public health concern. This Web site will answer many of your questions about ADD (AD/HD) and will direct you to other reliable sources online. The site is a work in progress, and some pages are still under construction . . . so we encourage you to bookmark the page and return often. New information and updates will be posted regularly.

www.help4adhd.org

Patricia O. Quinn, MD, Director, National Center for Girls and Women with AD/HD

3268 Arcadia Place, NW
Washington, DC 20015
www.ncgiadd.org
www.addvance.com

Sites for Coaches and Organizers

A.D.D. Resource Center

The A.D.D. Resource Center provides proven, practical tools and strategies to help individuals with attention-deficit hyperactivity disorder and related disorders to succeed.

www.addrc.org

ADHD Coaches Organization (ACO)

ACO is the professional membership organization for ADHD coaches. It is committed to serving as a resource for ADHD coaches, for its members and for the public. ACO is a nonprofit association created to advance the profession of ADHD coaching worldwide.

www.adhdcoaches.org

American Coaching Association

P.O. Box 353
Lafayette Hill, PA 19444
Telephone: (610) 825-4505
www.americoach.org

Edge Foundation

The Edge Foundation provides coaches for high school and college students with ADHD.

www.edgefoundation.org

Nancy Ratey
www.nancyratey.com

National Association of Professional Organizers (NAPO)
www.napo.net

Terry Matlen
www.addconsults.com

Sites for Women and Girls With ADHD

• www.adddiva.com	Web site for women with ADHD
• www.ADDFibro.com	Web site created by a woman diagnosed with ADD and fibromyalgia who offers a few articles and links to other Web sites
• www.facebook.com/ ADHDMoms	Social networking site for moms of children with ADHD
• www.flylady.com	Web site with great organizing tips
• www.gogirlsclub.org	Web site for girls with ADHD; a part of ADHDaware.org
• www.LivingwithADD.com	A private Web site offering articles, personal stories, books, audiotapes, gadgets, and organizing tips
• www.momswithadd.com	Private Web site with resources for moms with ADHD
• www.ncgiadd.org	National Center for Girls and Women with AD/HD
• www.sarisolden.com	Personal Web site of one of the leading experts on women with ADD (ADHD)

Bibliography and Additional Readings of Interest

Abikoff, H., McGough, J., Vitiello, B., McCracken, J., Davis, M., Walkup, J. et al. (1999). Sequential pharmacotherapy for children with comorbid attention-deficit/hyperactivity and anxiety disorder. *Journal of the American Academy of Child and Adolescent Psychiatry, 38*, 402–409.

ADDvance Magazine. (1997). How to form a women's support group. *ADDvance Magazine: A Magazine for Women With Attention Deficit Hyperactivity Disorder, 1*(2), 27.

Adelizzi, J. (2002). Posttraumatic stress in women with AD/HD. In P. O. Quinn & K. N. Nadeau (Eds.), *Gender issues and AD/HD: Research, diagnosis and treatment* (pp. 365–393). Washington, DC: Advantage Books.

American Academy of Child and Adolescent Psychiatry. (2002). Practice parameter for the use of stimulant medications in the treatment of children, adolescents, and adults. *Journal of the American Academy of Child and Adolescent Psychiatry, 41*, 26S–49S.

American Academy of Pediatrics. (2001). Clinical practice guidelines: Diagnosis and evaluation of the child with attention-deficit/hyperactivity disorder. *Pediatrics, 105*, 1158–1170.

American Psychiatric Association. (1994). *Diagnostic and statistical manual of mental disorders* (4th ed.). Washington, DC: Author.

American Psychiatric Association. (2000). *Diagnostic and statistical manual of mental disorders* (4th ed., text rev.). Washington, DC: Author.

American Psychiatric Association. (2010). *DSM-5: Options being considered for AD/HD.* Washington, DC: Author.

Arcia, E., & Conners, C. K. (1998). Gender differences in AD/HD? *Journal of Developmental and Behavioral Pediatrics, 19*, 77–83.

Arnold, L. E. (1996). Sex differences in AD/HD: Conference summary. *Journal of Abnormal Child Psychology, 24*, 555–569.

Arnold, L. E. (2001). Alternative treatments for adults with attention-deficit hyperactivity disorder (AD/HD). *Annuals of the New York Academy of Sciences, 931*, 310–341.

Arnold, L. E. (2002). Treatment alternatives for attention-deficit/hyperactivity disorder. In P. J. Jensen & J. Cooper (Eds.), *Attention-deficit/hyperactivity disorder: State of the science and best practices.* Kingston, NJ: Civic Research Institute.

Arnold, L. E., & DiSilvestro, R. A. (2005). Zinc in attention-deficit/hyperactivity disorder. *Journal of Child and Adolescent Psychopharmacology, 15*, 619–627.

Arnold, L. E., Kleykaml, D., Votolato, N., Gibson, R. A., & Horrocks, L. (1994). Potential link between dietary intake of fatty acids and behavior: Pilot exploration of serum lipids in attention-deficit hyperactivity disorder. *Journal of Child and Adolescent Psychopharmacology, 4*, 171–182.

Arpels, J. C. (1996). The female brain hypoestrogenic continuum from the premenstrual syndrome to menopause: A hypothesis and review. *Journal of Reproductive Medicine, 41,* 633–639.

Barkley, R. A. (1994). Personal communication at NIMH Sex Differences Conference, reported in Arnold, L. E. (1996). Sex differences in AD/HD: Conference summary. *Journal of Abnormal Child Psychology, 24,* 555–568.

Barkley, R. A. (1995). Sex differences in AD/HD. *AD/HD Report, 3,* 1–4.

Barkley, R. A., Murphy, K., & Fischer, M. (2007). *AD/HD in adults: What the science says.* New York, NY: Guilford Press.

Baumrind, D. (1971). Current patterns of parental authority. *Developmental Psychology Monograph, 4,* 1–103.

Biederman, J. (1998). Attention-deficit/hyperactivity disorder: A life-span perspective. *Journal of Clinical Psychiatry, 59,* 4–16.

Biederman, J., Ball, S. W., & Monuteaux, M. C. (2007). Are girls with AD/HD at risk for eating disorders? Results from a controlled, five-year prospective study. *Journal of Developmental and Behavioral Pediatrics, 28,* 302–307.

Biederman, J., Faraone, S. V., Mick, E., Williamson, S., Wilens, T. E., Spencer, T. J. et al. (1999). Clinical correlates of AD/HD in females: Findings from a large group of girls ascertained from pediatric and psychiatric referral sources. *Journal of the American Academy of Child and Adolescent Psychiatry, 38,* 966–975.

Biederman, J., Faraone, S., Spenser, T., Wilens, T., Norman, D., Lapey, K. A., et al. (1993). Patterns of psychiatry comorbidity, cognition, and psychosocial functioning in adults with attention deficit hyperactivity disorder. *American Journal of Psychiatry, 150,* 1792–1798.

Biederman, J., Mick, E., Bostic, J. Q., Prince, J., Daly, J., Wilens, T. E. et al. (1998). The naturalistic course of pharmacologic treatment of children with manic-like symptoms: A systemic chart review. *Journal of Clinical Psychiatry, 59,* 628–637.

Biederman, J., Mick, E., & Faraone, S. (2000). Age-dependent decline of symptoms of attention deficit disorder: Impact of remission, definition, and symptom type. *American Journal of Psychiatry, 157,* 816–818.

Biederman, J., Monuteaux, M.C., Mick, E., Spencer, T., Wilens, T. E., Klein, K. L. et al. (2006). Psychopathology in females with attention-deficit/hyperactivity disorder: A controlled, five-year prospective study. *Biological Psychiatry, 60,* 1098–1105.

Bloch, M. H., Panza, K. E., Landeros-Weisenberger, A., & Leckman, J. F. (2009). Meta-analysis: Treatment of attention-deficit/hyperactivity disorder in children with comorbid tic disorders. *Journal of American Academy of Child and Adolescent Psychiatry, 48,* 884–893.

Briscoe-Smith, A. M., & Hinshaw, S. P. (2006). Linkages between child abuse and attention-deficit/hyperactivity disorder in girls: Behavioral and social correlates. *Child Abuse and Neglect, 30,* 1239–1255.

Resources

Brown, R. T., Freeman, W. S., Perrin, J. M., Stein, M. T., Amler, R.W., Feldman, H. M. et al. (2001). Prevalence and assessment of attention-deficit/hyperactivity disorder in primary care settings. *Pediatrics, 107,* e43.

Brown, T. E. (1998, October). *AD/HD in persons with superior IQs: Unique risks.* Presented at the 10th Annual CHADD International Conference, New York, NY.

Burton, L. (2005). *AD/HD, gender-role discrepancy, and well-being in adult women* (PhD dissertation). Fielding Graduate University, Santa Barbara, CA.

Castellanos, F. X., Giedd, J. N., Elia, J., Marsh, W. L., Ritchie, G. F., Hamburger, S. D. et al. (1997). Controlled stimulant treatment of AD/HD and comorbid Tourette's syndrome: Effects of stimulant and dose. *Journal of the American Academy of Child and Adolescent Psychiatry, 36,* 589–596.

Chang, K. D., Steiner, H., & Ketter, T. A. (2000). Psychiatric phenomenology of child and adolscent bipolar offspring. *Journal of the American Academy of Child and Adolescent Psychiatry, 39,* 453–460.

Chronis-Tuscano, A., Seymour, K. E., Stein, M. A., Jones, H. A., Jiles, C.D., Rooney, M. E. et al. (2008). Efficacy of osmotic-release oral system (OROS) methylphenidate for mothers with attention-deficit/hyperactivity disorder (AD/HD): Preliminary report of effects on AD/HD symptoms and parenting. *Journal of Clinical Psychiatry, 69,* 1938–1947.

Cohen, C. (2000). *How to raise your child's social IQ.* Washington, DC: Advantage Books.

Conners, C. K. (1994). Personal communication at NIMH Sex Differences Conference, reported in Arnold, L. E. (1996). Sex differences in AD/HD: Conference summary. *Journal of Abnormal Child Psychology, 24,* 555–568.

Cortese, S., Konofal, E., Lecendreux, M., Arnulf, I., Mouren, M. C., Darra, F. et al. (2005). Restless legs syndrome and attention-deficit/hyperactivity disorder: A review of the literature. *Sleep, 28,* 1007–1013.

Diamond, I. R., Tannock, R., & Schachar, R. J. (1989). Response to methylphenidate in children with AD/HD and comorbid anxiety. *Journal of the American Academy of Child and Adolescent Psychiatry, 28,* 882–887.

Dukarm, C. (2005). Bulimia nervosa and ADD: A possible role for stimulant medication. *Journal of Women's Health, 14,* 345–350.

Dukarm, C. (2006). *Pieces of a puzzle: The link between eating disorders and ADD.* Washington, DC: Advantage Books.

Eiraldi, R., Cohen, I., Marshall, S., & Power, T. (2006, October). *Impairment in girls with subthreshold AD/HD.* Poster presentation, CHADD Conference, Chicago, IL.

Faraone, S. V., & Biederman, J. (1994). Is attention deficit hyperactivity disorder familial? *Harvard Review of Psychiatry, 1,* 271–287.

Faraone, S. V., Biederman, J., Mennin, J., Wozniak, J., & Spencer, T. (1997). Attention deficit hyperactivity disorder with bipolar disorder: A familial subtype? *Journal of the American Academy of Child and Adolescent Psychiatry, 36,* 1378–1387.

Faraone, S. V., Biederman, J., & Mick, E. (2006). The age-dependent decline of attention deficit disorder: A meta-analysis of follow-up studies. *Psychological Medicine, 36,* 159–165.

Faraone, S. V., Biederman, J., Spencer, T., Wilens, T., Seidman, L. J., Mick, E. et al. (2000). Attention-deficit/hyperactivity disorder in adults: An overview. *Biological Psychiatry, 48,* 9–20.

Feingold, B. F. (1985). *Why your child is hyperactive.* New York, NY: Random House.

Fellman, W. (2006). *Finding a career that works for you: A step-by-step guide to choosing a career.* Plantation, FL: Specialty Press.

Findling, R., Short, E., McNamara, N., Demeter, C. A., Stansbury, R. J., Gracious, B. L. et al. (2007). Methylphenidate in the treatment of children and adolescents with bipolar disorder and attention-deficit/hyperactivity disorder. *Journal of the American Academy of Child and Adolescent Psychiatry, 46,* 1445–1453.

Froehlich, T. E., Lanphear, B. P., Epstein, J. N., Barbaresi, W. J., Katusic, S. K., & Kahn, R. S. (2007). Prevalence, recognition, and treatment of attention-deficit/hyperactivity disorder in a national sample of U.S. children. *Archives of Pediatric and Adolescent Medicine, 61,* 857–864.

Gaub, M., & Carlson, C. L. (1997). Gender differences in AD/HD: A meta-analysis and critical review. *Journal of the American Academy of Child and Adolescent Psychiatry, 36,* 1036–1045.

Geller, B., & Luby, J. (1997). Child and adolescent bipolar disorder: A review of the past 10 years. *Journal of the American Academy of Child and Adolescent Psychiatry, 36,* 1168–1176.

Geller, T., Donnelly, C., Lopez, F., Rubin, R., Newcorn, J., Sutton, V. et al. (2007). Atomoxetine treatment for pediatric patients with attention-deficit/hyperactivity disorder with comorbid anxiety disorder. *Journal of the American Academy Child and Adolescent Psychiatry, 46,* 1119–1127.

Gershon, J. (2000). A meta-analytic review of gender differences in AD/HD. *Journal of Attention Disorders, 5,* 143–154.

Glod, C. A., & Teicher, M. H. (1996). Relationship between early abuse, post-traumatic stress disorder, and activity levels in prepubertal children. *Journal of the American Academy of Child and Adolescent Psychiatry, 34,* 1384–1393.

Greenhill, L., Kollins, S., Abikoff, H., McCracken, J., Riddle, M., Swanson, J. et al. (2006). Efficacy and safety of immediate-release methylphenidate treatment for preschoolers with AD/HD. *Journal of the American Academy of Child and Adolescent Psychiatry, 45,* 1284–1293.

Harris Interactive Poll. (2008). *Adult AD/HD.*

Harvey, E., Danforth, J. S., McKee, T. E., Ulaszek, W. R., & Friedman, J. L. (2003). Parenting of children with attention-deficit/hyperactivity disorder (AD/HD): The role of parental AD/HD symptomatology. *Journal of Attention Disorders, 7,* 31–42.

Resources

211

Hinshaw, S. P. (2002). Preadolescent girls with attention-deficit/hyperactivity disorder: I. Background characteristics, comorbidity, cognitive and social functioning, and parenting practices. *Journal of Consulting and Clinical Psychology, 70,* 1086–1098.

Hinshaw, S. P., Carte, E. T., Sami, N., Treuting, J. J., & Zupan, B. A. (2002). Preadolescent girls with attention-deficit/hyperactivity disorder: II. Neuropsychological performance in relation to subtypes and individual classification. *Journal of Consulting and Clinical Psychology, 70,* 1099–1111.

Hinshaw, S. P., Owens, E. B., Sami, N., & Fargeon, S. (2006). Prospective follow-up of girls with attention-deficit/hyperactivity disorder into adolescence: Evidence for continuing cross-domain impairment. *Journal of Consulting and Clinical Psychology, 74,* 489–499.

Johnson, M., Östlund, S., Fransson, G., Kadesjö, B., & Gillberg, C. (2009). Omega-3/omega-6 fatty acids for attention deficit hyperactivity disorder: A randomized placebo-controlled trial in children and adolescents. *Journal of Attention Disorders, 12,* 394–401.

Justice, A. J., & deWit, H. (1999). Acute effects of d-amphetamine during the follicular and luteal phases of the menstrual cycle in women. *Psychopharmacology, 145,* 67–75.

Justice, A. J., & deWit, H. (2000). Acute effects of estradiol pretreatment on the response to d-amphetamine in women. *Neuroendocrinology, 71,* 51–59.

Katz, L. J., Goldstein, G., & Geckle, M. (1998). Neuropsychological and personality differences between men and women with AD/HD. *Journal of Attention Disorders, 2,* 239–247.

Kessler, R., Adler, L., Barkley, R., Biederman, J., Conners, C. K., Demler, O. et al. (2007). The prevalence and correlates of adult AD/HD in the United States: Results from the national comorbidity survey replication. *American Journal of Psychiatry, 163,* 716–723.

Klingberg, T., Fernell, E., Olesen, P., Johnson, M., Gustafsson, P., Dahlstrom, K., et al. (2005). Computerized training of working memory in children with AD/HD—A randomized, controlled trial. *Journal of the American Academy of Child and Adolescent Psychiatry, 44,* 177–186.

Krause, K. H., Krause, J., Magyarosy, I., Ernst, E., & Pongratz, D. (1998). Fibromyalgia syndrome and attention deficit hyperactivity disorder: Is there a co-morbidity and are there consequences for the therapy of fibromyalgia syndrome? *Journal of Musculoskeletal Pain, 6,* 111–116.

Lahey, B. B., Applegate, B., McBurnett, K., Biederman, J., Greenhill, L. L., Hynd, G. W. et al. (1994). DSM-IV field trials for attention deficit disorder in children and adolescents. *American Journal of Psychiatry, 151,* 1673–1685.

Lithman, J., & Rodin, G. (2002). Fibromyalgia/chronic fatigue in women with AD/HD. In P. O. Quinn & K. G. Nadeau (Eds.), *Gender issues and AD/HD:*

Research, diagnosis and treatment (pp. 302–352). Washington, DC: Advantage Books.

Littman, E. (2009). *Toward an understanding of the AD/HD-trauma connection.* Retrieved from www.drellenlittman.com/ARTICLES.html.

March, J. S., Swanson, J. M., Arnold, L. E., Hoza, B., Conners, C. K., Hinshaw, S. P. et al. (2000). Anxiety as a predictor and outcome variable in the multimodal treatment study of children with AD/HD (MTA). *Journal of Abnormal Child Psychology, 28,* 527–541.

Mayes, S. D., Calhoun, S. L., & Crowell, E. W. (2000). Learning disabilities and AD/HD: Overlapping spectrum disorders. *Journal of Learning Disabilities, 33,* 417–424.

McCann, D., Barrett, A., Cooper, A., Crumpler, D., Grimshaw, K., Kitchin, E. et al. (2007). Food additives and hyperactive behavior in 3-year-old and 8/9-year-old children in the community: a randomised, double-blinded, placebo-controlled trial. *The Lancet, 370,* 1560–1567.

McGee, R., Williams, S., & Feehan, M. (1992). Attention deficit disorder and age of onset of problem behaviors. *Journal of Abnormal Child Psychology, 20,* 487–502.

Michelson, D., Read, H. A., Ruff, D. D., Witcher, J., Zhang, S., & McCracken, J. (2007). CYP2D6 and clinical response to atomoxetine in children and adolescents with AD/HD. *Journal of the American Academy of Child and Adolescent Psychiatry, 46,* 242–251.

Mikami, A. Y., Hinshaw, S. P., Patterson, K. A., & Lee, J. C. (2008). Eating pathology among adolescent girls with attention-deficit/hyperactivity disorder. *Journal of Abnormal Psychology,117,* 225–235.

Millstein, R., Wilens, T., Biederman, J., & Spencer, T. (1997). Presenting symptoms of AD/HD in clinically referred adults with AD/HD. *Journal of Attention Disorders, 2,* 159–166.

Monastra, V. J., Lubar, J. F., & Linden, M. (2001). The development of a quantitative electroencephalographic scanning process for attention deficit-hyperactivity disorder: Reliability and validity studies. *Neuropsychology, 15*(1), 136–144.

Murray, C., & Johnston, C. (2006). Parenting in mothers with and without attention-deficit/hyperactivity disorder. *Journal of Abnormal Psychology, 155,* 52–61.

Nadeau, K. G. (1997). *ADD in the workplace: Choices, changes and challenges.* Bristol, PA: Brunner/Mazel.

Nadeau, K. G. (2002). Neurocognitive psychotherapy for women with AD/HD. In P. O. Quinn & K. G. Nadeau (Eds.), *Gender issues and AD/HD: Research, diagnosis and treatment.* (pp. 220–254). Washington, DC: Advantage Books.

Nadeau, K. G. (2004). *Does your gifted child have ADD/AD/HD?* Retrieved from http://www.addvance.com/help/parents/gifted_child.html.

Resources

Nadeau, K. G., Littman, E. B., & Quinn, P. O. (2001). *Understanding girls with ADD*. Washington, DC: Advantage Books.

Nora, J. J., Vargo, T. A., Nora, A. H., Love, K. E., & McNamara, D. G. (1970). Dextroamphetamine: A possible environment trigger in cardiovascular malformation. *Lancet, 1*, 1290–1291.

Ohan, J., & Johnson, C. (2005). Gender appropriateness of symptom criteria for attention-deficit/hyperactivity disorder, oppositional defiant disorder and conduct disorder. *Child Psychiatry and Human Development, 35*, 359–381.

Ohan, J., & Visser T. (2009). Why is there a gender gap in children presenting for attention deficit/hyperactivity disorder services? *Journal of Clinical Child and Adolescent Psychology, 38*, 650–660.

Owens, J. (2005). The AD/HD and sleep conundrum: A review. *Journal of Developmental and Behavioral Pediatrics, 26*, 312–322.

Owens, J. (2009). Neurocognitive and behavioral impact of sleep-disorder breathing in children. *Pediatric Pulmonology, 44*, 417–422.

Perry, B. D., & Pollard, R. (1998). Homeostasis, stress, trauma, and adaptation. *Child and Adolescent Psychiatry Clinics of North America, 7*, 33–51.

Quinn, P. O. (2002). Hormonal fluctuations and the influence of estrogen in the treatment of women with AD/HD. In P. O. Quinn & K. G. Nadeau (Eds.), *Gender issues and AD/HD: Research, diagnosis and treatment* (pp. 183–199). Washington, DC: Advantage Books.

Quinn, P. O. & Nadeau, K. N. (2002). *Gender issues and AD/HD: Research, diagnosis and treatment*. Washington, DC: Advantage Books.

Quinn, P. O., & Nadeau, K. G. (2006). *When moms and kids have ADD* (expanded version). Washington, DC: Advantage Books.

Quinn, P., & Wigal, S. (2004). Perceptions of girls and AD/HD: Results from a national survey. *MedGenMed, 6*, 2. Retrieved from http://www.medscape.com/viewarticle/472415.

Rabiner, D. L., Anastopoulous, A. D., Costello, J., Hoyle, R., & Swartzwelder, H. S. (2008). Adjustment to college in students with AD/HD. *Journal of Attention Disorders, 11*, 689–699.

Ramsay, J. R., & Rostain, A. (2005). Adapting psychotherapy to meet the needs of adults with attention-deficit/hyperactivity disorder. *Psychotherapy: Theory, Research, Practice and Training, 42*, 72–84.

Ratey, J. (2008). *Spark: The revolutionary new science of exercise and the brain*. New York, NY: Little, Brown and Company.

Richardson, W. (1997). *The link between ADD and addictions: Getting the help you deserve*. Colorado Springs, CO: NavPress.

Richardson, W. (2002). Addictions in women with AD/HD. In P. O. Quinn & K. G. Nadeau (Eds.), *Gender issues and AD/HD: Research, diagnosis and treatment* (pp. 394–410). Washington, DC: Advantage Books.

Richardson, W. (2005). *When too much isn't enough: Ending the destructive cycle of AD/HD and addictive behavior.* Colorado Springs, CO: Pinon Press.

Robison, R. J., Reimherr, F. W., Marchant, B. K., Faraone, S. V., Adler, L. A., & West, S. A. (2008). Gender differences in two clinical trials of adults with attention-deficit/hyperactivity disorder: A retrospective data analysis. *Journal of Clinical Psychiatry, 69,* 213–217.

Rucklidge, J. J., & Kaplan, B. J. (1997). Psychological functioning of women identified in adulthood with attention-deficit/hyperactivity disorder. *Journal of Attention Disorders, 2,* 167–176.

Rucklidge, J. J., & Tannock, R. (2001). Psychiatric, psychosocial, and cognitive functioning of female adolescents with AD/HD. *Journal of the American Academy of Child and Adolescent Psychiatry, 40,* 530–540.

Sachs, G. S., Baldassano, C. F., Truman, C. J., & Guille, C. (2000). Comorbidity of attention deficit hyperactivity disorder with early- and late-onset bipolar disorder. *American Journal of Psychiatry, 157,* 466–468.

Safren, S. A., Otto, M. W., Sprich, S., Winett, C. L., Wilens, T. E., & Biederman, J. (2005). Cognitive-behavioral therapy for AD/HD in medication-treated adults with continued symptoms. *Behaviour Research and Therapy, 43,* 831–843.

Schredl, M., Alm, B., & Sobanski, E. (2007). Sleep quality in adult patients with attention deficit hyperactivity disorder (ADHD). *European Archives of Psychiatry amd Clinical Neuroscience, 257,* 164–168.

Shekim, W. O., Asarnow, R. F., Hess, E., Zaucha, K., & Wheeler, N. (1990). A clinical and demographic profile of a sample of adults with attention deficit disorder-residual type. *Comprehensive Psychiatry, 31,* 416–425.

Sherman, C. (2003). Treating comorbid bipolar disorder and AD/HD. *Clinical Psychiatry News, 31,* 18.

Sherman, K. F. (2000). *A housekeeper is cheaper than a divorce: Why you CAN afford to hire help and how to get it.* Mountain View, CA: Life Tools Press.

Sobanski, E., Schredl, M., Kettler, N., & Alm, B. (2008). Sleep in adults with attention deficit hyperactivity disorder (AD/HD) before and during treatment with methylphenidate: A controlled polysomnographic study. *Sleep, 31,* 375–381.

Solden S. (1995). *Women with attention deficit disorder: Embracing disorganization at home and in the workplace.* Grass Valley, CA: Underwood Books.

Solden, S. (1997). Ask Sari. *ADDvance Magazine, 1*(2), 12.

Sonuga-Barke, E. J., Daley, D., & Thompson, M. (2002). Does maternal AD/HD reduce the effectiveness of parent training for preschool children's AD/HD? *Journal of the American Academy of Child and Adolescent Psychiatry, 41,* 696–702.

Spencer, T., Biederman, J., Wilens, T., Harding, M., O'Donnell, D., & Griffen, S. (1996). Pharmacotherapy of attention deficit disorder across the life cycle. *Journal of the American Academy of Child and Adolescent Psychiatry, 35,* 409–432.

Resources

Spencer, T., Biederman, J., Wilens, T., Prince, J., Gerard, K., Doyle, R. et al. (2001). Efficacy of a mixed amphetamine salts compound in adults with attention-deficit/hyperactivity disorder, *Archives of General Psychiatry, 58,* 775–782.

Spencer, T., Wilens, T., Biederman, J., & Faraone, S. (1995). A double-blind, crossover comparison of methylphenidate and placebo in adults with childhood onset attention deficit hyperactivity disorder. *Archives of General Psychiatry, 52,* 434–443.

Stein, M. A., Sandoval, R., Szumowski, E., Roizen, N., Reinecke, M. A., Blondis, T. A. et al. (1995). Psychometric characteristics of the Wender Utah rating scale (WURS): Reliability and factor structure for men and women. *Psychopharmacology Bulletin, 31,* 423–431.

Stephens, P. (2010). *Reversing chronic disease: A journey back to health.* Mustang, OK: Tate Publishing.

Surman, C. P., Adamson, J. J., Petty, C., Biederman, J., Kenealy, D. C., Levine, M. et al. (2009). Association between attention-deficit/hyperactivity disorder and sleep impairment in adulthood: Evidence from a large controlled study. *Journal of Clinical Psychology, 70,* 1523–1529.

Surman, C., Randall, E., & Biederman, J. (2006). Is there an association between AD/HD and bulimia? *Journal of Clinical Psychiatry, 67,* 351–354.

Szatmari, P. (1992). The epidemiology of attention-deficit hyperactivity disorder. *Child and Adolescent Psychiatric Clinics of North America, 1,* 361–371.

Taylor, A., & Kuo, F. (2009). Children with attention deficits concentrate better after walk in the park. *Journal of Attention Disorders, 12,* 401–409.

Turgay, A., Ansari, R., & Schwartz, M. (2006). Comorbidity differences in AD/HD throughout the life cycle. *Program and Abstracts of the American Psychiatric Association.* Toronto, Canada: American Psychiatric Association.

Tzelepis, A., Schubiner, H., & Warbasse, L. H. (1995). Differential diagnosis and psychiatric co-morbidity patterns in adult attention deficit disorder. In K. G. Nadeau (Ed.), *A comprehensive guide to attention deficit disorder in adults.* New York, NY: Brunner/Mazel.

Walker, C. (1999, May). *Gender and genetics in AD/HD: Genetics matter; gender does not.* Paper presented at the ADDA conference, Chicago, IL.

Weber, D. A., & Reynolds, C. R. (2004). Clinical perspectives on neurobiological effects of psychological trauma. *Neuropsychology Review, 14,* 115–129.

Weden, S., & Culotta, V. (2009). Sports participation and anxiety in children with AD/HD. *Journal of Attention Disorders, 12,* 499–506.

Weinstein, C. S., Apfel, R. J., & Weinstein, S. R. (1998). Description of mothers with AD/HD with children with AD/HD. *Psychiatry, 61,* 12–19.

Weinstein, D., Staffelbach, D., & Biaggio, M. (2000). Attention-deficit hyperactivity disorder and posttraumatic stress disorder: Differential diagnosis in childhood sexual abuse. *Clinical Psychology Review, 20,* 359–378.

Weiss, M., & Murray, C. (2003). Assessment and management of attention-deficit hyperactivity disorder in adults, *Canadian Medical Association Journal, 168,* 715–722.

Wilens, T. (2004). Impact of AD/HD and its treatment on substance abuse in adults. *Journal of Clinical Psychiatry, 65,* 38–45.

Wilens, T. E., Biederman, J., Brown, S., Tanguay, S., Monuteaux, M. C., Blake, C. et al. (2002). Psychiatric comorbidity and functioning in clinically referred pre-school children and school-aged youths with AD/HD. *Journal of the American Academy of Child and Adolescent Psychiatry, 41,* 262–268.

Wilens, T. E., Biederman, J., & Spencer, T. J. (2002). Attention-deficit/hyperactivity disorder across the lifespan. *Annual Review of Medicine, 53,* 113–131.

Wilens, T. E., Spencer, T. J., & Biederman, J. (1995). Are attention-deficit hyperactivity disorder and the psychoactive substance use disorders really related? *Harvard Review of Psychiatry, 3,* 260–262.

Wilens, T. E., Spencer, T. J., & Biederman, J. (2001). A review of the pharmacotherapy of adults with attention-deficit/hyperactivity disorder. *Journal of Attention Disorders, 5,* 189–202.

Wilens, T. E., Biederman, J., Spencer, T. J., & Prince, J. (1995). Pharmacotherapy of adult attention-deficit/hyperactivity disorder: A review. *Journal of Clinical Psychopharmacology, 15,* 270–279.

Wolraich, M. L., Wilson, D. B., & White, J. W. (1995). The effect of sugar on behavior or cognition in children: A meta-analysis. *Journal of the American Medical Association, 274,* 1617–1621.

Wood, P. B. (2004). Stress and dopamine: Implications for the pathophysiology of chronic widespread pain. *Medical Hypotheses, 62,* 420–424.

Young, J. L. (2002). Depression and anxiety in women with AD/HD. In P. O. Quinn & K. G. Nadeau (Eds.), *Gender issues and AD/HD: Research, diagnosis and treatment* (pp. 270–291). Washington, DC: Advantage Books.

Young, J. L. (2007). *AD/HD grown up: A guide to adolescent and adult AD/HD.* New York: W. W. Norton.

Zak, R., Fisher, B., Convadelli, B. V., Moss, N. M., & Walters, A. S. (2009). Preliminary study of the prevalence of restless legs syndrome in adults with attention deficit hyperactivity disorder. *Perceptual Motor Skills, 108,* 759–763.

Zylowska, L., Acherman, D. L., Yong, M. H., Futrell, J. L., Horton, N. L., Hale, T. S. et al. (2008). Mindfulness meditation training in adults and adolescents with AD/HD: A feasibility study. *Journal of Attention Disorders, 11,* 737–746.

Resources

Glossary

A

Adderall: A psychostimulant medication made up of amphetamine salts. Indicated for the treatment of the symptoms of ADHD.

Addiction: A chronic neurobiologic disorder that has genetic, psychosocial, and environmental dimensions and is characterized by one of the following: the continued use of a substance despite its detrimental effects, impaired control over the use of a drug (compulsive behavior), and preoccupation with a drug's use for nontherapeutic purposes (i.e., craving the drug).

ADHD-addiction: The link between ADHD and the development of various addictions.

ADHD coach: A lifestyle coach who has a special understanding of ADHD issues who can work in a relationship with persons with ADHD to help them achieve short- and long-term goals.

ADHD-friendly lifestyle: A lifestyle in which the person with ADHD

works with his strengths instead of struggling against his weaknesses.

Aerobic exercise: Any physical exercise that increases the heart rate and over time increases cardiovascular fitness.

Alternative therapies: Treatments other than medication and behavioral interventions (psychosocial intervention) that treat the symptoms of ADHD with an equally or more effective outcome.

American Psychiatric Association (APA): The APA is the major professional organization for psychiatrists in the United States.

Amphetamine: A psychostimulant used to treat ADHD that increases attention and the ability to concentrate while decreasing hyperactivity and distractibility.

Anorexia: The symptom of not feeling hungry, often resulting in decreased appetite.

Anorexia nervosa: An eating disorder that usually involves excessive weight loss and is accompanied by a distorted body image and drive for thinness.

Anticonvulsants: Medications used to treat seizures.

Antidepressants: Medications used to treat depression.

Arrhythmia: Any abnormal electrical activity in the heart.

Atomoxetine: A nonstimulant medication used in the treatment of ADHD that is a norepinephrine reuptake inhibitor. The trade name of atomoxetine is Strattera.

Attention span: A person's attention span is the amount of time that he or she is able to concentrate on any one thing. It usually increases with age.

Authoritarian parenting style: Parenting style in which the parents are usually demanding and make most or all of the decisions for a child.

Authoritative parenting style: Parenting style in which the parents are both demanding and responsive.

B

Behavior management: Psychosocial treatment for ADHD involving both positive and negative reinforcement to change behavior.

Binge eating: A pattern of disordered eating that consists of periods during which a person consumes a quantity of food that is greater than that which is usually consumed in one sitting.

Bipolar mood disorder (BMD): A mental health disorder characterized by a history of one or more episodes of mania, or abnormally elevated mood, and intermittant periods of depressive mood separated by periods of normal mood.

Blood pressure (BP): BP is the force that is exerted by blood circulating on the blood vessel walls. It is measured both when the heart pumps (systolic blood pressure) and between beats (diastolic blood pressure) and is written in mm of mercury (Hg) as one value over the other (SBP/DBP), such as 130/65 mmHg.

Brain scans: Noninvasive procedure that is done to image the anatomy and function of the brain. Brain scans use several techniques including CAT (computerized axial tomography), MRI (magnetic resonance imaging), and SPECT (single photon emission computed tomography) scans.

Breakthrough seizure: Seizures that occur during control with medication.

Bright light therapy: A treatment involving exposure to bright, full-spectrum light for a specific amount of time to regulate sleep–wake cycles and to treat seasonal affective disorder.

Bulimia nervosa: An eating disorder defined as binge eating followed by purging behaviors including self-induced vomiting, the use of laxatives, or, more rarely, the use of diuretics.

C

Cardiac defect: A defect in the structure of the heart.

Chemical neurotransmitter: Chemical released from a nerve cell in order to relay signals within the nervous system.

This process is commonly described as a lock-and-key phenomenon.

Chronic fatigue syndrome: A debilitating disorder defined by persistent fatigue unrelated to exertion and not substantially relieved by rest, and accompanied by the presence of other specific symptoms for a minimum of 6 months.

Classroom trauma: A significantly unpleasant external event or stressor, occurring within the confines of an educational environment that is usually psychological in nature.

Clinically significant impairment: Impairment that places the patient outside the range of normal functioning.

Clonidine: A medication used to treat several medical conditions, including high blood pressure. It has also been used as an off-label treatment for ADHD.

Coaching: A method of training a person or group of people to improve performance or specific skills.

Coexisting condition: Additional major or minor condition that co-occurs with another medical or mental health disorder.

Cognitive behavioral therapy (CBT): A psychotherapeutic approach that uses goal-oriented, directive therapy to change internal scripts to deal with maladaptive behaviors and emotions.

Cognitive deficit: This term describes any characteristic or quality that negatively affects intellectual performance or ability, whether it is genetic or caused by one's environment (the normal aging process, neurologic disorders, brain injuries, and mental illness).

Concentration: The ability to focus and pay attention.

Concerta: A long-acting stimulant medication that delivers methylphendate over 12 hours by using osmotic-release technology.

Conduct disorder: A mental health disorder marked by a pattern of aggressive or antisocial behaviors such as cruelty toward people and pets, lying, truancy, vandalism, and stealing.

Congenital: Present from birth.

Continuous performance test: An objective neurophysiologic measure of attention. Continuous performance tests measure the subject's response to computer-generated stimuli where errors of omission (indicating degree of inattention) and commission (indicating degree of impulsivity); and an overall rate of variability of response times are obtained.

Criterion: One of a set of variables required to define a condition or disorder.

D

Daydreaming: Divergent thoughts, plans, or fantasies experienced while awake.

Deep breathing: Taking deep breaths in and out using the lungs, diaphragm, and abdominal muscles rather than the muscles of the rib cage only.

Demoralization: The destruction of one's morale or disheartenment.

Depression: A mood disorder characterized by feelings of sadness, helplessness, and hopelessness.

Dexedrine: An amphetamine and one of the stimulant medications used to treat ADHD. It is twice as potent as the other class of stimulants (methylphenidate).

Diagnostic and Statistical Manual of Mental Disorders **Fourth edition, Text Revision (DSM-IV-TR):** Published by the American Psychiatric Association, this text is the primary tool for diagnosis of mental disorders.

Diverticulum (plural: diverticula): An outpouching of a hollow or fluid-filled structure in the body.

Dopamine: One of the chemical transmitters in the brain that functions by stimulating the receptors on nearby cells.

Dyad: A pair.

Dysphoria: An unpleasant or uncomfortable mood.

Dysthymia: Chronic low-level depression.

E

Eating disorder: An eating disorder is marked by a pattern of abnormal eating ranging from insufficient to excessive food intake.

Echocardiogram: A sonogram of the heart.

Effective dose: The amount of a medication that produces a reduction in symptoms in the majority of people taking it.

Electroencephalogram: The recording of electrical activity within the brain as measured by electrodes placed on the scalp.

Emotional dysregulation: A poorly regulated emotional response, commonly referred to as a mood swing.

Estradiol: The predominant sex hormone present in females.

Estrogen: The female sex hormone.

Executive function: One of the primary functions of the frontal lobes of the brain. This brain process allows for initiating, planning, strategizing, and inhibiting activities.

External locus of control: A person's belief that factors beyond his control (such as chance, fate, or others) determine events in his life.

F

Family meeting: Meetings held at regular intervals within the home involving all family members to discuss issues, problem solve, and make plans.

Family tree: A chart representing family relationships.

Fibromyalgia: A chronic pain disorder, its symptoms include musculoskeletal pain, fatigue, sleep disturbance, and joint stiffness.

Field trial research: Research conducted to determine the parameters of a certain disorder.

First-line treatment: The first and usually most effective medication used to treat a certain condition.

Focalin: One of the stimulant medications used to treat ADHD, containing only the active isomer of methylphenidate.

G

Gender-role expectations: Expected behaviors that are assigned based on a person's gender.

Gene: The basic unit of heredity.

Generalized anxiety disorder: A mental health disorder marked by excessive and irrational worry that is out of proportion to the source of the worry and interferes with daily functioning.

Genetic test: A test for risk factors that can indicate possibility of inheriting certain diseases.

Growth: An increase in height or weight over time.

Growth retardation: Smaller than expected height and weight for age.

Guanfacine: A long-acting drug that is used to treat ADHD, its brand names include Tenex and extended release Intuniv.

H

Heart rate: The number of times the heart beats per minute.

Hormone: Chemical released by the cells in a gland that affects other cells in the body.

Hormone replacement therapy: The use of synthetic or natural hormones to replace those that are deficient.

Hot flash: The flushing, sweating, and overheating that is a symptom of the changing hormone levels that go along with menopause.

Hyperactivity: Purposeless motor activity that is more than expected developmentally.

Hyperreactive: Uncontrollably reactive to stimuli.

Hypersensitivity: Overly sensitive to stimuli.

Hypertalkative: Excessively talkative.

Hypothyroidism: Condition resulting from the underproduction of the thyroid hormone.

I

Imaging studies: Procedures that produce an image of parts of the body for the purpose of diagnosis of a medical condition.

Impairment: A disability in a certain area of functioning.

Impulsivity: Acting without thinking.

Inattentive: Not paying attention.

Indulgent parenting style: Parenting style practiced by parents who allow their children to do whatever they wish.

Inherited: Condition that is passed down by genetic transmission.

Insomnia: A sleep disorder resulting in persistent difficulty falling asleep and/or staying asleep.

Internalize symptoms: Condition where feelings are directed inward towards the self.

Intelligence quotient (IQ): A person's IQ is a score derived from a standardized test whose function is to evaluate intelligence.

Glossary

223

L

Learned helplessness: Behavior that results from the feeling that one has little or no control over the outcome of a situation.

Learning disability: A disorder in which a person has difficulty learning. May involve reading, math, or written expression.

Long-acting stimulant: Medication that lasts 6 to 12 hours after taking just one dose.

M

Major depression: A mental health disorder marked by feelings of hopelessness, low self-esteem, and loss of interest in normally enjoyable activities; and can also include changes in eating and sleeping habits.

Mania: An episode of abnormally elevated energy levels and/or mood that can also involve grandiosity and other expansive behaviors.

Meditation: An activity whereby a person enters into a state of relaxation or inner awareness.

Melatonin: A natural chemical in the body whose levels change to follow a daily cycle.

Menopause: A stage in the female reproductive cycle, traditionally indicated by the permanent stopping of monthly menstruation, ending fertility.

Menstrual cycle: The monthly cycle of physiological changes (including the blood flow) that occurs in females.

Methylphenidate: A stimulant medication used for treatment of ADHD. It is the main component in Ritalin, Methylin, Metadate, and Concerta.

Mood stabilizers: Various medications used in the treatment of mood disorders including the mania and depression associated with bipolar disorder.

Multimodal treatment: A program utilizing several forms of interventions or treatments.

N

National survey: A large-scale survey or study to determine the prevalence or rates of a condition or opinions.

Negligent parenting style: Style of parenting in which parents provide only for their child's basic needs, but are not supportive or encouraging. They often fail to monitor and supervise activities.

Neonatal withdrawal: Symptoms seen in an infant after birth (poor feeding, crying, and irritability) as a result of exposure to an addicting substance before birth.

Neurobiologic: Anything that pertains to the biology of the nervous system.

Neurotransmitter: Chemicals that send signals between brain cells.

Nonpharmacologic: Therapies involving techniques or specialized programs, herbs, special diets, or various supplements other then medication.

Nonstimulant medication: Medications for the treatment of ADHD that are not stimulants.

Norepinephrine: A chemical that affects the sympathetic nervous system and acts as a neurotransmitter.

O

Obsessive-compulsive disorder (OCD): An anxiety disorder marked by intrusive thoughts (obsessions) and the need to perform certain behaviors (compulsions). A person with OCD will usually develop rituals and various other repetitive behaviors in order to decrease anxiety.

Obsessive-compulsive personality disorder (OCPD): OCPD is a personality disorder (whereas OCD is an anxiety disorder) that is characterized by obsessions with perfection, rules, and organization that are usually targeted in a specific area. A person with this disorder will usually develop routines and rules for ways of doing things and has difficulty allowing others to take on tasks for fear they will not do them as well as he or she can do them.

Obstructive sleep apnea (OSA): A sleep disorder seen in adults and children involving pauses in breathing while sleeping that is caused by airway obstruction.

Off-label: Use of a medication for a condition for which it is not approved.

Omega-3 fatty acid: An essential fatty acid found in cold water fish, flax, and nuts.

Oppositional behavior: Stubborn, defiant behavior.

Oppositional defiant disorder (ODD): An ongoing pattern of disobedient, hostile, and defiant behavior toward authority figures that goes beyond the bounds of normal childhood behavior.

Organizational skills: Skills that enable someone to be organized and efficient.

Overactive: Excessive motor activity, but with a purpose.

P

Parenting style: A set of characteristic behaviors and strategies that parents use in their child-rearing.

Perimenopause: The years before menopause during which the production of hormones (including estrogen, progesterone, and testosterone) decreases resulting in the onset of symptoms of menopause.

Premature birth: Infant born before 37 weeks gestation.

Premenstrual dysphoric disorder (PMDD): Severe premenstrual symptoms that can be debilitating including severe irritability and depressed mood.

Premenstrual syndrome (PMS): The group of symptoms (physical, psychological, and emotional) seen prior to a woman's period that can cause discomfort and impair functioning.

Preschooler: A child before formal education, usually between the ages of 3 and 5 years.

Prevalence rate: The rate of occurrence of a disease in a population.

Professional organizer: A person who helps individuals and businesses develop a plan to organize their surroundings.

Progesterone: A hormone whose level increases during the latter part of the menstrual cycle or pregnancy.

Progressive muscle relaxation: This technique involves tensing and relaxing muscles in a systematic way to reduce anxiety.

Provigil: Provigil, the brand name for modafinil, increases alertness and can be used to treat shift-work sleep disorder, narcolepsy, and excessive daytime sleepiness resulting from obstructive sleep apnea.

Psychosis: A state of mind that involves a break from reality and may include auditory or visual hallucinations.

Psychosocial treatment: Interventions that specifically address problems that a person might have with social skills and certain behaviors.

Psychotherapy: Sessions held with a counselor or a psychotherapist that address problems with day-to-day functioning.

Psychotherapy group: A form of therapy in which at least one therapist meets with and treats a small number of clients as a group.

Puberty: A stage in development involving physical and hormonal changes that cause a child's body to become an adult's body.

R

Rapid-cycling bipolar mood disorder: Specific subgroup of bipolar disorder in which a person has four or more episodes of mania or depression per year.

Rating scale: A set of questions used to get information about the presence of symptoms of a disorder or state that can be used to objectify subjective behaviors and determine severity.

Recovery: Process of recovering from an injury or illness.

Reframing: A technique that helps a person to see things more positively or from another point of view (frame) so that he or she may feel better about the situation.

Restless legs syndrome (RLS): A condition that is characterized by an irresistible urge to move one's legs or other body parts in order to stop uncomfortable or odd sensations.

Ritalin: The brand name of the stimulant medication methylphenidate that is used for the treatment of attention-deficit hyperactivity disorder.

S

School phobia: The presence of extreme stress or other emotional or learning problems that can bring about a refusal to attend school.

Second-line therapy: Medication that is used as a second choice to treat a disorder.

Seizure: Abnormal electrical activity in the brain that can cause a change in mental state, tonic or clonic movements, or convulsions.

Self-esteem: Overall estimation of one's self-worth.

Self-regulation: The ability to control one's emotions and behaviors through the executive functions.

Sensory integration dysfunction: Difficulty with processing and organizing sensory information as it comes into the brain.

Sex-based norm: Norm or criterion based on the gender of the person.

Sex-linked condition: A disorder in which the gene that causes it is located on the X or Y chromosome.

Sexual intimacy: Sexual intercourse.

Short-acting stimulant: Immediate release medication that becomes effective in a short time and lasts up to 4 hours.

Side effect: A harmful or undesired effect that occurs as a result of using a medication.

Sleep apnea: A disorder marked by breathing pauses during sleep.

Sleep disorder: Abnormal sleep patterns that may be seen in both adults and children and involve the inability to fall or stay asleep.

Stimulants: Class of medications used to treat ADHD that reduce hyperactivity and impulsivity and improve attention span.

Stress analysis: Taking a look at or making a list of what is causing one's stress.

Substance abuse: The overuse of or dependence on a drug that causes negative effects on a person's physical or mental health.

Subthreshold: A condition where symptoms are present, but below the level or number needed to formally meet the criteria to make a diagnosis.

Support group: Group where members provide each other with various insights and help. Members are usually not professionals and often share or identify with a common condition, diagnosis, or disease.

T

Thyroid hormone: Chemical produced by the thyroid gland and involves the use of iodine.

Tic: A sudden, repetitive, stereotyped motor movement or vocalization involving specific muscle groups.

Time-out: A behavior management technique for disciplining a child. May also be used as a time to retreat and get oneself together.

Total treatment program: Program to treat ADHD involving several different forms of therapy including medication, education, and psychosocial treatments.

Tourette's syndrome: A congenital disorder marked by the presence of multiple motor tics, including at least one vocal tic. In addition, the person may demonstrate symptoms of problems with learning and attention, and obsessive-compulsive traits.

Toxic mother/daughter dyad: An unhealthy relationship between a mother and her daughter with ADHD, where the mother is typically hypercritical and the daughter is oppositional.

Trauma: A physical, emotional, or psychological injury, usually resulting

Glossary

227

from an extremely stressful or life-threatening situation.

V

Vegetative symptom: Inability to eat or sleep or excessive sleeping, usually associated with depression.

Verbal memory: Memory of what is said.

Vitamin supplement: A preparation intended to provide vitamins that are missing in a person's diet.

Vyvanse: The brand name for a stimulant that combines phenethylamine with an amphetamine. It is used to treat ADHD and has a lower abuse potential than other amphetamines because of its unique properties.

W

Wellbutrin: Wellbutrin, the brand name for bupropion, works as an atypical antidepressant and can also be used to help people quit smoking.

Word retrieval: The ability to recall a word from memory.

Y

Yoga: A form of exercise that combines stretching, physical movements, postures, and deep breathing to improve concentration and deepen relaxation. Yoga may also be considered a form of meditation.

Index

Index

seizures
  breakthrough, 83
  uncontrolled, 87
self-esteem
  ADHD and, in women/girls,
    25–27
  CBT for, 88–89
  dating and, 140
  of girls, 25–27
  low, 11
  of men, 26
  promotion of, 62
sensory integration dysfunction, 139
  ADHD and, 51–52
  dealing with, 52–53
sexual intimacy, ADHD and,
  138–139
shame
  criticism and, 61
  in girls, 48
  treatment of, 59
shopping addiction, 34
short-acting stimulants, 137
side effects
  common types of, 83
  insomnia as, 82
  of stimulants, 83
sleep apnea, 168
sleep disorders
  ADHD and, 164–168
  in adults, 168
  patterns of, 39
  restless, 165
  of women, 164
social skill issues
  with ADHD, 126–128
  in girls, 126–129
  parents' involvement with, 127
societal stereotypes, 19–21
sound, adjusting to, 51–52
St. John's Wort, 93
stereotypes, societal, 19–21
stimulants
  anxiety from, 86
  BMD and, 87
  BP and, 84
  cardiac conditions and, 84
  contraindications to, 86–87
  effectiveness of, 68–69
  glaucoma and, 86
  insomnia and, 82
  long-acting, 137
  mania and, 87
  during pregnancy, 86

short-acting, 137
side effects of, 83
tics and, 86
Tourette's syndrome and, 86
Strattera (atomoxetine), 44, 65, 67
stress
  ADHD and, 132–134
  in adolescence, 60
  analysis of, 132
  management of, 133
  in marriage, 145–146
substance abuse, in girls, 24
supervisors, relationship with, 119–120
supplementation
  nutrition and, 92–93
  with vitamins, 137
support groups
  benefits of, 100
  for girls, 59–60
  tips for, 101

T

teachers
  symptom recognition by, 14–15
  understanding of, 176
Tenex (guanfacine), 64
therapists, 134
three-breath technique, 91
thyroid hormone, 137
tics, 73
  stimulants and, 86
time management
  breaking cycle of, 102–103
  changes in, 15
  in college, 177
  problems with, 106
  strategies for, 107
  tips for, 104–105
time-out, emotional, 61
Tofranil (imipramine), 67
touch, adjusting to, 51
Tourette's syndrome, stimulants and, 86
toxic relationship, 47
trauma, ADHD and, 45–46
treadmill, 96

U

unfinished projects, 111–112

V

vegetative symptoms, 72
verbal memory, 136
vitamin supplements, 137
Vyvanse (lisdexamfetamine), 64, 67